Healing Glaucoma

Natural Medicine for Self-Healing

Glen Swartwout

A.B., B.D., O.D., N.D., F.I.C.A.N., F.C.S.O.

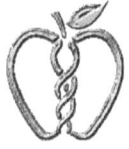

Published by Healing Oasis

Hilo, Kingdom of Hawai'i

Titles by Rev. Dr. Glen Swartwout

Refreshing Vision: Opening the Windows of the Soul

Cataract Solutions: Prevention & Reversal Via Accelerated Self-Healing

Healing Glaucoma

Macular Degeneration... ...Macular Regeneration

Dry Eye Relief: Natural Medicine for Accelerated Self-Healing

The Shire: Cultivating Your Future Self

Materia Medica: Vis Medicatrix Naturae

Anima Medica: Vis Medicatrix Naturae

Electromagnetic Pollution Solutions

Biofields: The New Physics of Health

Nous Energy: Healing Power of the Pyramids

As Above, So Below: The Coherence of All Creation

The Living Universe: A Fractal Hologram

Free E-zine signup: http://tryUnity.net

DVDs by Rev. Dr. Glen Swartwout

A Clinical Theory of Everything

The Five Phases of Disease

The Five Phases of Healing

The Five Tissue Layers

The Five Levels of Regulation

The Five Elements of Spiritual Development

The Hard Question of Consciousness

The Arrow of Time

"This book is a great contribution to the emerging paradigm of 21st century vision care. It provides a thorough review of many healing modalities in order to help a person's eye, body and soul heal the condition of glaucoma... A must for any patient or professional working with this condition. Dr. Swartwout is a pioneer in helping to regenerate our precious gift of sight."

- Marc Grossman, O.D., L.Ac.
Co-author of Greater Vision
Co-author of Natural Eye Care

Table of Contents

Foreword

If you are reading this book as a patient, self-healer or caregiver seeking answers beyond those offered by your eye doctor, I am glad that you are here on the threshold of what I hope and pray will be a most productive journey of learning, exploring and healing for you... not only for your eyes and your vision, but for your life... in all the many aspects that go into a complete picture of health, and a sense of purpose, meaning and direction in life. After all, not only are healthy eyes important to serve the essential function of vision, but improving and safeguarding our vision is important to serve the sentient life of our consciousness, our mind, our soul.

Vision is ultimately a core function of our true selves as navigational spiritual beings, not merely a biophysical transduction of photons to electrical nerve current, though that is the foundation upon which we learn to derive meaning from the select visible octave of frequencies of quantum energy that is also the source of most biological energy itself, received from the sun, and captured in all the covalent bonds of carbon chemistry that constantly reconstructs the standing waves that are these bodies through which we experience the gift that is this life.

If you are a practitioner of the healing arts, congratulations! I applaud the openness of your mind, and your heart's unfettered motivation for seeking out answers for healing those souls who put their faith and trust in your guidance, wherever that quest may lead you... It is a sacred trust, which we should hold dear. Never allow the pressures for human respect by your peers, nor for worldly treasure sway you from seeking truth, and offering it freely to those who can hear. The riches you will store in Heaven's true economy of sacred gifts will enrich your own spirit, and the lives of all you touch. My father, who was also a pioneering eye doctor in the fields of functional, behavioral and developmental optometry, told me when I first began to practice with him, "You have learned a lot, enough to start practicing... Listen to your patients. They will teach you the rest." He was a good doctor, and a wise man who had practiced what he preached. His admonition beats the usual warning given physicians in medical school: "Don't listen to your patients. They have no medical training. They will throw you off track..."

I am still listening to each person who seeks my guidance, and after thirty years, I am still amazed at the rich tapestry from which to learn from the unique experiences and observations of each human being in the process of living, learning, growing and healing... from the intricacies of the body's inner linguistics to the transcendent gestalt of unique personhood that hovers beyond words... from the flavor of each personality, unique from conception, to the radiant sense of overarching coherence between the biological challenges of the living vessel, and the psycho-emotional life of the conscious spirit itself, the ghost within the machine of life, that is the reason we seek a deeper way of healing!

Preface

This book has been growing over the years... contributed to in various stages as I began researching the relationship between vision and nutrition when I opened my first professional practice in 1982, the Optometric Center of Tokyo. I interned with a number of leading nutritionally oriented Doctors of Optometry including Conrad Mazeski, Don Getz, Ben Lane, Moses Albalas and Robert Kaplan. I was asked to speak to an international meeting of the International College of Applied Nutrition, of which I was a Fellow, and this stimulated the beginnings of formalizing and organizing my thinking and knowledge base in this vitally important, relatively untapped area of health care. The individualized clinical application of natural methods for accelerating self-healing of eye diseases such as glaucoma remains in its infancy three decades later. My hope is that this introductory guide and reference book can help those who are called to explore and pioneer this fertile terrain for the benefit of future generations.

Introduction

This book is offered as a tour guide, a sort of black book survey of potential solutions that have already proven useful for others seeking outside the paradigmatic box of modern conventions in med-surge medicine, for how the body can heal in the face of glaucoma.

These solutions have worked for many people in my healing practice over the past three decades, and they have worked for me personally. Without them, I would have been expected to be blind for the past decade or so. Not only have I retained my vision without eye drops or surgical intervention, I have experienced the side benefits of hundreds of non-toxic, natural therapies designed to improve other supportive body functions over the years to achieve this. Eyes do not get sick... or well... in a vacuum. Eyes depend upon nutrients to function properly and repair themselves. Nutrients are supplied to the eyes by the digestive system via the circulatory system, pumped by the heart, oxygenated by the lungs, cleansed by the liver and kidneys, and wastes are drained by the lymph system, and the list goes on...

The most efficient way to healthier eyes, and the healing of the underlying causes of glaucoma, is to heal the whole person, one step at a time, according to the priorities identified by the body's own healing and communication systems. Fortunately, we now have methods to tap into this communication system, more or less like hooking up a modern car to a diagnostic computer. And through the holographic nature of the body's design, we can do that non-invasively, through electrodermal measurements of the body's purposeful responses to signals, the same kind of signals the body itself uses for internal regulation. This is new language of the body's biological energy field, or biofield, allows me to ask directly whether a given tissue is calling out in distress, and whether a particular medicine carries the signature of healing energy it can utilize to complete its mission for healing that distress. This is a process which is ongoing in the body every second we are alive... It's just now that we are beginning to learn how to listen...

"Eye pressure at Hawaiian Eye Clinic: 42 & 46. One month later, eye pressure at Hawaiian Eye Clinic: 30 & 31 without using any eye drops or chemical drugs. Used only herbal caps of Forskohlii" noted Dr. Kuakiniokalani Keeaumoku Kawananakoa-Prible, His Serene Highness, Hawaiian Prince and European Royal who grew up in Buckingham Palace.

The ophthalmologist at Hawaiian Eye, the #1 eye clinic in Hawaii, had prescribed eye drops, which he had informed Dr. Kuakini he did not expect to work. He was amazed at the reduced eye pressures, thinking that the prescription had worked.

When Dr. Kuakini informed him that he had not filled the prescription, since he was told they would not work anyway, but had instead taken an herbal remedy, the ophthalmologist was even more amazed and said that it was the first time he had ever seen a natural substance reduce a patient's eye pressure.

Dedication

This volume in my eye health solution series is dedicated to Dr. Schuyler McCulloch Martin, an early pioneer in hospital based research on vitamin nutrition, and energy medicine, having worked with Steinmetz at General Electric.

Dr. Martin, for whom I am named, was our family physician as I was growing up. He had saved my Grandmother from DDT poisoning, and had identified my intolerance of cow's milk, referring my parents to the nearest goat farm for milk that I could digest, due to the much smaller size of proteins in goat milk compared to the casein in cow's milk. We will never know the problems we have prevented at a level of primary prevention, but like my grandma, I probably owe him my life...

Glaucoma Solutions

Glaucoma actually represents many different diseases, affecting all age groups from newborns to the elderly. It can be very painful, or can progress without any symptoms. Glaucoma is a major cause of irreversible blindness. Glaucoma is often associated with high pressure in the eyes, however a high percentage of people with glaucoma have normal or even low pressure. Ultimately, the final cause of vision loss in each type of glaucoma is an inability to get the needed nutrients to the cells of the retina and optic nerve, as well as to remove metabolic wastes and any other toxins that may be present in these tissues of the central nervous system.

Medical and surgical controls of intraocular pressure are sometimes necessary and should be utilized when less invasive means of management alone are insufficient. Drugs and surgery appear to suppress glaucoma damage only for a limited time for each individual, though. Drugs and surgery do not correct or eliminate the underlying causes of disease, which are always individual and typically multi-factorial. Learning more about your biochemical individuality and how to be a good steward of your body are necessary in order to achieve your optimum potential for health and longevity.

As many as 15 million Americans may have glaucoma, of which 1.6 million already suffer some loss of vision, and over a quarter million are blinded by it in at least one eye. The cost is over $2.5 billion each year, mostly for medical and surgical care, including over 7 million office visits. With the aging of our population, these figures are rapidly increasing, despite the fact that 50% of glaucoma continues to go undiagnosed. Even in diagnosed cases, 70% of the vision loss occurs prior to diagnosis, despite the fact that 47% have been examined by an ophthalmologist or optometrist within one year prior to diagnosis.

Loss of optic nerve fibers occurs well before any change can be detected in visual fields. With increased use of general practitioners as gatekeepers in managed care, this situation may worsen, since 78.4% of primary care practitioners falsely believe intraocular pressure (IOP) is the only diagnostic indicator of glaucoma. In truth, most people with elevated IOP, an estimated 7 million Americans, have ocular hypertension, 80% of whom never develop detectable signs of glaucoma, though they do lose 25 to 40% of the 1,200,000 nerve cells in the optic nerve.

At the same time, 60% of those with glaucoma have normal or even low pressure in the eye. Glaucoma can occur at pressures as low as 12, while the optic nerve can sustain pressures as high as 24 without damage. The common category of low-tension glaucoma, which can be associated with hypertension, diabetes, migraines, cold extremities and heart disease, is thought to be caused by vasoconstriction, and 30% of cases appear to show optic nerve damage from systemic causes including anemia, heart disease and hypertension.

Glaucoma is actually a constellation of collagen-vascular diseases (i.e. connective tissue and blood vessel conditions related to processes like rheumatoid arthritis and atherosclerosis), which cause similar types of peripheral vision loss. The Cardiovascular Health Center at Harvard concludes that non-pharmacological approaches to cardiovascular diseases should be the first method of treatment by physicians.

Atherosclerotic plaque

The trabecular meshwork shows Endothelial Leukocyte Adhesion Molecule-1 (ELAM-1), the first step in atherosclerotic plaque formation, in glaucoma of diverse etiology (Nature Med 2001, 7:304-309). ELAM-1 is controlled by an interleukin-1 autocrine feedback loop. Damage to the lining of the outflow pathway triggers transcription factor NF-kappaB, which then stimulates release interleukin-1, other inflammatory cytokines, and ELAM-1.

About 90% of glaucoma cases are of the insidious primary open angle type involving constricted blood flow and nutrition to the optic nerve with either normal (15 to 21 mm Hg) or elevated pressure (over 21 mm Hg). About 10% consist of low-pressure (less than 15 mm Hg) glaucoma, which also involves decreased ocular blood flow. More rare types of glaucoma include the typically painful but periodic acute angle closure type as well as pigmentary, inflammatory and congenital glaucomas. Together, the glaucomas represent the second greatest cause of blindness in America, with 70,000 affected to the point of blindness.

Pseudo-Exfoliation

Pseudo-Exfoliation (PEX) Syndrome is risk factor for glaucoma, found in 6-12% of open angle glaucoma, more in the elderly and in women. Drug treatments include beta blockers and prostaglandins, while surgeries used are laser trabeculoplasty and trabeculotomy.

Pseudo-Exfoliation is linked to Alzheimer's, senile dementia, cerebral atrophy, chronic cerebral ischemia, stroke, TIA's, heart disease, and hearing loss. PEX is associated with abnormal extracellular matrix and basement membrane structural protein functions. Resultant protein deposits could theoretically be remediated by oral proteolytic enzymes, especially taken on an empty stomach to maximize systemic absorption as is done for treatment of inflammation and pain. Other natural anti-inflammatory therapies may also be useful. PEX is more common in Scandinavians due to the LOXL1 gene for enzyme linking intracellular collagen & elastin.

High homocysteine associated with Pseudo-Exfoliation can be recycled into functional SAMe by methyl donors, especially TMG and MSM.

Low ascorbate in PEX can be remedied by supplemental vitamin C and assisted by bioflavonoids, with HMC Hesperiden especially indicated to stabilize mast cell membranes to reduce allergy related

4

causal chains. Vitamin C may also help prevent stress from the high energy photons in sunlight. Vitamin C is specifically concentrated in the aqueous humor, and effectively acts as a UV filter. PEX is also associated with high malondialdehyde and 8-iso-prostaglandinF2a.

Autoimmune contributions to PEX suggest the use of immune modulators such as phytosterols. These would help with immunity against viral components also seen in some cases.

Collagen

What all these conditions have in common is not elevated intraocular pressure (IOP), but morphological changes in the collagen structure of the lamina cribrosa (the part of the sclera or white connective tissue layer of the eye through which the optic nerve passes), the papillary blood vessels (which provide nutrition to the papilla, or optic nerve head, where it passes through the lamina cribrosa), and the trabecular meshwork (the filter through which the eye fluid, or aqueous humor, passes to reach Schlemm's canal, the drainage channel which removes fluid from the eye and delivers it back into the blood vessels).

Even in glaucoma cases where pressure does become elevated, causing further risk of damaging the optic nerve fibers (axons), the connective tissue changes precede the changes in IOP. In most cases of glaucoma, vision loss occurs with these micro-structural changes even without an increase in IOP.

Glaucoma may be an extension of myopia (nearsightedness, involving stretching of the sclera), which occurs when the elastic limit of the sclera is exceeded by the intraocular pressure, thus causing expansion at the optic nerve (a change in shape called "cupping") with resulting loss of vascular flow and neuronal function. Both glaucoma and myopia are associated with other collagen disorders, including Ehlers-Danlos syndrome, Marfan's syndrome, and osteogenesis imperfecta.

One study of the systemic health of glaucoma patients found that 30% had low-tension glaucoma, 42% had high tension glaucoma and 28% had identifiable systemic causes including anemia, carotid obstruction, syphilis and intracranial tumor.

Large diurnal fluctuations in IOP during the day or over consecutive days, such as those associated with food sensitivity and allergy are associated with an increased risk of glaucoma progression over and above more traditional risk factors such as age, race and sex. (Asrani S, Zeimer R, Wilensky J, et al. Large diurnal fluctuations in intraocular pressure are an independent risk factor in patients with glaucoma. J Glaucoma. 2000; 9: 134-42.) Diurnal pressures of normal subjects vary by only 3.7 mm Hg, while medically treated glaucoma patients still show 7.6 mm Hg variation compared to untreated patients with 11 mm Hg variation. (Drance SM. Diurnal variation of intraocular pressure in treated glaucoma: significance in patients with chronic simple glaucoma. Arch Ophth. 1963; 70: 302-11. Drance SM. The significance of diurnal tension variation in normal and glaucomatous eyes. Arch Ophth. 1960; 64: 494-501.)

The Advanced Glaucoma Intervention Study found that patients whose pressure was 18 mm Hg or lower at every visit over 6 years had almost no progressive visual field loss. (The AGIS Investigators. The Advanced Glaucoma Intervention Study (AGIS): 7. The relationship between control of intraocular pressure and visual field deterioration. Am J Ophthalmol 2000; 130(4): 429-40.)

In a more recent study, medical patients with a low daily IOP variance as well as low minimum and maximum IOP had the lowest probability of developing a new visual field defect over a 5-year period. Subjects treated with Travatan (a PGF 2 derivative) had the lowest average IOP and the lowest variance as compared with the other treatment groups. (Nordmann JP, LePen C, Berdeaux G. Estimating the long-term visual field consequences of average daily intraocular pressure and variance. Clin Drug Invest 23(7): 431-438. 2003.)

Forskolin (Colforsin) works on the complementary IOP-lowering but anti-inflammatory PGE 2 pathway via the cAMP-mediated EP 2, EP 3 and EP 4 receptors. A rational beginning approach to glaucoma prevention therapy is to monitor IOP regularly at several times of day using the home eye pressure monitor while following a rotation diet to identify and eliminate food triggers of IOP elevation spikes and supplementing with oral Forskolin, Omega-3 fatty acids: EPA & DHA plus other IOP regulating (e.g. Melatonin at night for morning pressure spikes) and neuroprotective supplements, especially L-Carnosine, as indicated clinically and/or by resonance matching using energetic biofeedback. Drinking microwater and rebounding are also central to a balanced anti-glaucoma lifestyle. The target IOP is a daily maximum of 15 to 18 with a diurnal variability of up to 3 mm Hg. In the same embryonic tissue layer as the connective tissue is the circulatory system. Circulation, both lymphatic and vascular, seems to be a real key to understanding and preventing glaucoma. When looking at circulatory patterns among glaucoma patients, two types of problems emerge. In one group, there is vasoconstriction, causing symptoms like cold hands. In the second distinct group, the problems relate to blood clotting, resulting in symtoms like electrocardiogram (ECG) abnormalities. The risk factors that affect glaucoma are generally those associated with vascular problems, including hypertension, hypotension, migraine, increased blood viscosity, carotid artery stenosis, heart disease, and even a familial tendency, which is true of vascular disease in general. Vascular abnormalities have been confirmed in every type of glaucoma via Doppler ultrasound. Optic disc hemorrhages are commonly seen several years before glaucoma is diagnosed, and they undoubtedly occur but go undetected in many additional cases. Dilated and tortuous retinal blood vessels are also frequently seen in the retina, and these have been linked to coronary artery disease. Loss of optic nerve fibers is directly related to decreased pumping ability of the heart. Severe loss of visual fields are seen in 42% of glaucoma patients, but 70% of those with atrial fibrillation have severe losses. Atrial fibrillation is also twice as likely among glaucoma patients as compared to normals. Decreased blood flow to the eyes causes structural changes over time that result in increased IOP. Glaucoma patients have narrowed retinal blood vessels compared to normals. Thermography, such as used in the new field of Ophthermology, shows that 89% of glaucoma patients have cerebral vascular disease! Computed tomography (CT) has shown that 90.3% of low-tension glaucoma patients have calcification of the carotid artery near the opening of the optic canal, as compared to only 20.8% of individuals the same age, but without glaucoma. Magnetic resonance imaging (MRI) shows deep white matter lesions in the brain in low-tension glaucoma patients, another effect of reduced cranial blood flow. Low-tension glaucoma is also associated with peripheral and central vasoconstriction (e.g. migraine) and spontaneous blood clots. Blood clot formation is more common in glaucoma patients compared to those with ocular hypertension, and low-tension glaucoma patients show higher blood viscosity than those with high-tension glaucoma. Blood flow measurements taken in the fingers of low-tension glaucoma patients shows rates significantly below normal. 44% of low-tension glaucoma patients suffer classic migraine symptoms and in elderly sufferers of low-pressure glaucoma this figure can be as high as 86%. Silent heart attacks (myocardial ischemia) is found in 3% of 'normal' adults, but one study found 30.8% in low-tension glaucoma patients in a 24 hour period, which was double the rate found in both normal subjects and chronic open angle glaucoma. Stenosis of the carotid artery can be an underlying cause of symptoms diagnosable as glaucoma, and restoring carotid blood flow can temporarily increase and then normalize IOP. Increased blood viscosity (hematocrit above 50) is often found in glaucoma patients. This can impair blood flow when combined with elevated IOP.

Limits of Conventional Care

Drugs and Surgery

Medical and surgical treatments are actually aimed at lowering IOP rather than improving the underlying collagen metabolism. Among individuals with ocular hypertension (elevated IOP), only those who also show cupping appear to be at risk for visual field loss. Reversal of cupping changes is sometimes seen with filtering "bleb" surgery, but has not been shown with medical treatments. According to an extensive review of the medical literature, a 30% reduction in IOP is needed to reverse cupping, and this is why the IOP reduction from most medications is not clinically significant in changing the rate of progression of vision loss in glaucoma. Beta-blocker eye drops can reduce IOP somewhat (6 mm Hg, preventing further loss of peripheral vision for 3 to 6 years), but do not improve blood flow to the eyes. Medical treatment even fails to control IOP in most cases (53%) of glaucoma within just 4 years. Laser surgery fails to control IOP in 23% the first year and 70% after just 10 years. Over 50% have to take drugs treatments in addition after just 2 years. Glaucoma itself increases the risk of cataracts by 2.9 times, but when surgery is added, this jumps to 14.3 times increased risk.

Side effects of glaucoma drugs are a real problem, causing up to 62% to fail to follow the recommended treatment. Beta blocker drops commonly cause side effects including: low blood pressure, confusion, depression, dizziness, headache, impotence, hair loss, skin and nail changes, diarrhea, nausea, asthma, breathing difficulty, and increased LDL cholesterol. On average, glaucoma patients 'forget' to take their medication on 112 days each year. Patient surveys show that 30% experience side effects like changes in heart rhythm, congestive heart failure, and difficulty breathing. Hundreds actually die each year from respiratory problems caused by glaucoma drugs. One study also shows that 80% of glaucoma patients on beta-blocker drugs experience depression, compared to only 26% of patients with serious eye problems who do not take these drugs. Beta-blocker eye drops used for glaucoma have other serious implications for body chemistry. Timoptic, for example, reduces 'good' HDL cholesterol, while increasing 'bad' LDL cholesterol, enough to increase the risk of heart attack by 17%. Since heart attacks cause about half of all deaths in this country, this increased risk represents a major problem. When beta-blockers fail to control IOP, treatment with other drugs with even worse side effects may be considered, such as carbonic anhydrase inhibitors (e.g. acetazolamide), which, although they can increase blood flow to the retina, cause kidney problems, fatigue, lethargy, anorexia, weight loss, depression, dementia, loss of libido, and occasionally aplastic anemia. Drug treatment decisions are often based on visual field tests, which accurately show the progression of the disease only 43% of the time.

A comparable situation exist with blood pressure, another convenient functional measure which can be manipulated by pharmaceutical intervention. A study in England looked beyond the medical consensus that patients were healthier on medications because their BPs were reduced. The patients, their families and others in the community showed a very different consensus that health, energy, function and quality of life was reduced. The body is not a machine that can be best maintained with aftermarket parts. It is however, a self-regulating, self-healing vital organism adapted to be responsive to a broad array factors that have existed and continue to exist in our natural environment. Known traditionally as the Vis Medicatrix Naturae (the healing power of nature), it is the source of some 1/3 of our pharmaceuticals and the model for synthesis of perhaps another 1/3. The biggest limitation on natural healing is that there is so little money in it, lacking enforcement of monopoly pricing via patents, and licensing requirements demanded for harmful treatments. Given licensure requirements and standards of care, there is very little opportunity, other than an occasional case like mine of self treatment, for the exploration of nontoxic and noninvasive methods for healing conditions like glaucoma.

Many types of medical therapy can actually cause glaucoma. Corticosteroids in the form of eye drops, creams, pills, inhalers and injections are a common trigger, since these drugs polymerize molecules in the drainage system of the eye, while inhibiting the formation and repair of collagen and glycosaminoglycans (GAGs) necessary for maintaining normal structure and function of both the eye's lamina cribrosa and the trabecular meshwork. Steroidal eye drops, for example, increase glaucoma risk seven-fold. There is no safe level of corticosteroid use and even stopping or changing medication once IOP elevation occurs does not always solve the problem, since up to a third of these cases of induced glaucoma are irreversible with standard medical/surgical treatment leaving permanent damage to the optic nerve. Even creams for eczema and inhalers (with over 8 million annual prescriptions in America alone) can cause increased IOP. Corticosteroids increase oxidative stress, which impairs the phagocytic (debris clearing) ability of cells in the eye's drainage system.

Many over-the-counter drugs can trigger acute attacks of glaucoma in susceptible individuals. Drugs that chelate metal ions like zinc (e.g. diodohydroxyquin, iodochlorhydroxyquin and ethambutol) can cause optic nerve atrophy like that seen in glaucoma. Zinc supplementation is recommended preventively for all patients on such medications. Optic nerve toxicity is also known to occur with aspirin, ibuprofen, tranquilizers, antidepressants (e.g. lithium, MAO inhibitors), antibiotics (e.g. chloramphenicol, isoniazide, ethambutol), and medications for diabetes. Visual defects caused by this kind of toxicity are usually attributed to other causes, such as glaucoma. Even the preservatives used in many eye drops, including most glaucoma medications, may trigger chronic inflammation of the eye that can worsen glaucoma. Benzalkonium chloride used to preserve Timoptic, Betoptic,

Optipranolol, and Ocupress anti-glaucoma drops increases dry eye symptoms by 250%. Merck manufactures an unpreserved beta-blocker eye drop called OcuDose. While unpreserved 'artificial tear' eye drops used for temporary eye lubrication reduce the permeability of the corneal surface of the eye by 44%, those preserved with benzalkonium chloride actually increase this leakiness by 8%, disrupting the epithelial cell membrane that protects the integrity of the eye. The concentrations used, from .4 to 1 part per thousand (equivalent to a 3X homeopathic potency) are toxic to the cornea and, through accumulation in body tissues over time, have even been documented cause such severe corneal toxicity as to require a corneal transplant. Preservatives such as benzalkonium chloride and thimerisol used in contact lens solutions can also accumulate to toxic levels within soft contact lenses themselves, thus exposing the cornea whenever wearing the lens. The chronic inflammation and allergy responses triggered by such toxic chemicals can result in the deposition of inflammatory proteins in the drainage system of the eye, thus increasing IOP and contributing to the risk for glaucoma. Inflammation in the eye area may also reduce the quality of blood and lymph drainage from the eye, which can also impair outflow of fluid from inside the eye. It also increases free radical activity, which is probably the ultimate cause of damage to nerve cells in glaucoma. Glaucoma is not only associated with hypertension, but also with hypotension. Anti-hypertensive medications may compound this problem, often triggering low blood pressures during sleep. This may deprive the optic nerve head of needed oxygen, resulting in loss of visual fields. Cardiac events also double at diastolic pressures of 75 comparted to 85 mm Hg. At systolic pressures below 140 mm Hg, glaucoma patients show 4 times the rate of visual field deterioration. Most glaucoma patients who progressively lose vision have blood platelets that tend to clump together spontaneously. Many drugs can also precipitate an angle closure glaucoma attack. These include motion sickness patches, and antihistamines.

Natural Medicine for Healing Glaucoma

Let's begin the journey through the array of potential natural solutions, many of which are assured to be beneficial or even crucial in eventually eliminating, as much as feasible, the multi-factorial causality of the particular type of glaucoma, which is ultimately unique to the physiology and pathophysiology of each individual at a given time in the progression of the disease and its potential reversal.

Risk Factors

Risk Factor Modification

The most significant controllable risk factors according to one report are untreated hypertension and cigarette smoking. Other major risk factors include free radical damage associated with aging, reduced health, hypotension, lack of exercise, poor nutrition, diabetes and other vascular diseases, as well as allergies and digestive problems. Other toxins that damage the optic nerve may be contributing factors in the loss of vision among glaucoma sufferers. These include tobacco, aspartame, methyl alcohol, and factors potentially present in blood transfusions, plus tea, coffee, and alcohol.

Coffee may increase cholesterol, resulting in reduced circulation to eye tissues, unless it is passed through a paper filter before consumption. While caffeine temporarily increases cerebral circulation, and does not increase IOP, it does promote vasospasms, which can contribute to glaucomatous vision loss. It also destabilizes blood sugar even more than refined sugar does, which is detrimental to nerve cell health. Caffeine promotes conversion of metallic mercury into methyl mercury and mercuric chloride by pathogenic fungi and bacteria. Both of these forms are approximately 1,000 times more toxic than the metal. In addition, Coffee impairs B12 absorption and destroys beneficial bacterial flora. On balance, the author recommends avoidance of coffee, other than possibly water process decaf green coffee for weaning off coffee, and diterpene and phenolic coffee extracts.

While some studies have found little relationship between smoking and glaucoma, one study showed a 2.9 times increased risk! Smoking constricts the internal lumen diameter of blood vessels and blocks the ability of vessels to redilate. After smoking a cigarette, vasoconstriction causes IOP to increase by more than 5 mm Hg in 37% of glaucoma patients and 11% of normals. Tobacco by itself can cause vision loss (tobacco amblyopia) as can alcohol (alcohol amblyopia), and can also contribute to nutritional deficiencies related to vision loss, by interfering with gastric production of hydrochloric acid and therefore preventing effective digestion and assimilation of many nutrients including vitamin B12. In some cases, supplemental vitamin B12 has reversed vision loss even despite continued smoking. Nicotine reduces retinal blood flow by 9.6 to 16.4% in diabetics who are at high risk for glaucoma as well as diabetic retinopathy. It is recommended that anyone who uses alcohol or tobacco should supplement at least 1500 to 3000 micrograms of vitamin B12, glutathione precursors such as cysteine and 600 I.U. of vitamin E to counteract the toxic effects of cyanide in the optic nerve as well as 1000 micrograms of folic acid. Folic acid has also been shown to improve visual acuity in smokers with optic neuropathy, with an average increase of 5 lines of visual acuity over a 2 month period! Supplementation of 300 milligrams of vitamin B1 weekly for 3 months by intramuscular injection (together with 1,000 micrograms of B12) has also been recommended for tobacco amblyopia.

Nicotine, LDL cholesterol and free radicals block acetylcholine receptors, increasing the tendency toward vasospasm. The vasomotor relaxation response to acetylcholine has been improved by lowering harmful LDL cholesterol levels. Some of the dietary means of accomplishing this include GTF Chromium, garlic, Vitamin C, onions, almonds, olive oil, fish oil, grape seed oil, and avocado, as well as antioxidants vitamin E and coenzyme Q10. This approach measurably increases the coronary artery diameter. This may also improve the ability of blood vessels to dilate in response to seratonin and aggregating platelets. Cigarette smoking is one of the major risk factors for glaucoma, along with hypertension (especially systolic), obesity and the amount of pigmentation in the iris. Blacks, having the greatest amount of pigmentation, have four times the risk of glaucoma and 8 times the risk of blindness from glaucoma compared to whites.

Familial patterns are often strong, as well, in all races, with relatives of a glaucoma victim being 20 times more likely to get glaucoma. This can be from hard-wired genetic patterns as well as from miasmatic inheritance transferred epigenetically, which eventually can be removed through homeopathy. Environmental factors are also very important, and have been found to play a strong role in exfoliation of the lens, which can cause ocular hypertension and triples the risk of glaucoma.

Such environmental effects are probably mediated via free radical pathology.

Obesity affects one out of three adults, the average weight having increased by 8 pounds between 1980 and 1991 to an average of 25 (female) to 30 pounds (male) overweight. Obesity increases blood pressure and secretion of adrenal hormones. In Japan, with the highest longevity in the world, overweight is not the norm, and IOP actually tends to decrease with age, the opposite of what is seen in America. In America, 8% of people over age 40 have increased IOP, and the rate of glaucoma climbs from 0.25% at age 20 to 1% at age 40 to 7% at age 70.

Lack of oxygen to the tissues in the eye can trigger neovascularization, which in turn can cause glaucoma. Oxygen therapies may also be helpful, along with electrons and other (nutritional) antioxidants and modalities to increase ocular blood flow, such as ginkgo.

Antiangioneogenesis factors present in shark and bovine cartilage may be beneficial in controlling or modulating this type of response, and were the first in this class to be explored clinically. The most potent antiangioneogenesis factor is found in bindweed (*Convulvulus arvensis* extract available clinically as Vascustatin), and additional antiangioneogenesis support can be accessed with Apigenin (4',5,7-trihydroxyflavone from celery, parsley and other vegetables and fruits), Coenzyme Q10, Diterpenes extracted from green coffee beans, Catechins extracted from *Camelia sinensis* (Green tea), Conjugated

Linoleic Acid (CLA), Curcumin from turmeric, Indole-3-Carbinol (I3C) from cruciferous vegetables like broccoli, Isoflavones extracted from soy, Lycopene from vine ripened tomatoes, Melatonin, N-Acetylcysteine (NAC), Oligomeric Proanthocyanidins (OPCs) extracted from grape seeds, Omega 3 fatty acids, Punicalagins (phenols made of carbohydrate bound ellagic acid, also called ellagitannins) extracted from pomegranate, Quercetin, Silibinin in Silymarin from milk thistle seeds, and Vitamin D.

Release of histamine and other pro-inflammatory substances seems to be a significant factor especially in low-tension glaucoma. 30% of low-tension glaucoma patients have immune-related problems, compared to only 8% of those with ocular hypertension. Immune complexes are extremely large molecules that tend to block outflow locally at the trabecular meshwork level, as well as downstream lymph nodes and the kidneys. Therapies to consider include the mast cell stabilizing bioflavonoid Hesperiden Methyl Chalcone (HMC), homeopathic Aller-Free and/or Food Tolerance, and a 7-day food allergy avoidance protein-sparing fast on a complete nutrition support like UltraBalance (from Metagenics), MediPro (from Thorne Research) or the author's favorite, One Step (from Progressive Labs), which he helped to inspire. Introducing foods can be reintroduced one per day while monitoring diurnal IOP oscillation with a ProView home IOP meter to detect IOP changes that may be caused by particular foods. Typical responses can be immediate or delayed up to 24 hours from exposure. Offending foods can then be eliminated completely from the diet, and other foods eaten on a rotation diet to minimize development of new reactions, which tend to be triggered when a food is consumed too regularly. For example, with candidiasis, the constant supply of a particular poorly digested food source will tend to induce *Candida albicans* to make epigenetic modifications in order to thrive on that food. Subsequently, attempts to avoid that food can trigger a Herxheimer, or die-off reaction, which clears upon eating the offending food, leading to cravings and an addictive cycle in which the candida's biocommunications can become confused and mistakenly identified as thoughts and desires of the host.

Laser treatments seem to be even less successful in glaucoma than are drugs. Laser may be most effective when used before any drug therapy is started, but most who have laser first still need drug treatment within 2 years. Surgery on the other hand is capable of increasing blood flow to the eye by 29%, but only in those who have not already started drug treatments. Surgery appears to have more potential benefits than conventional drug therapy in at least temporarily slowing the damage caused by glaucoma 3 to 6 times more effectively than laser or drugs, although not universally, nor without significant risks. Surgery is not effective at slowing the progression of glaucoma in the majority of cases represented by low-pressure glaucoma. Also, 15% of glaucoma surgery patients report a reduced quality of life following surgery, and 40% find no perceptible improvement. Surgery also needs to be repeated in many cases. Surgery of any kind is, by definition, controlled damage to the body, and such an invasive approach should be reserved whenever time permits until non-invasive methods have been exhausted. This follows the physician's oath "Primum non nocere," to above all do no harm.

The actual damage to nerve cells in the optic nerve, resulting in loss of vision, appears to be associated with hemorrhages of the blood vessels in the optic nerve head and related loss of cellular nutrition combined with free radical activity. Similar damage to the cells of the optic nerve is now known to occur during migraine headaches, when blood vessels constrict the flow of oxygen and other nutrients to the cells. The risk of developing measurable damage to the optic nerve goes up with increased IOP levels, from 15% at 24 mm Hg to 90% at 30 mm Hg, and nearly 100% at 33 mm Hg. Patients with healthy optic nerves and no peripheral vision loss can sustain pressures of 30 for up to 20 years without losing sight. Unfortunately, approximately 50% of the nerve cells in the optic nerve are lost before glaucomatous changes in the visual fields can be detected in an eye examination. This loss of nerve cells happens 2 to 6 years before changes show up on peripheral vision tests. Intervention in the presence of ocular hypertension and other risk factors has been shown to reduce the loss of peripheral vision and optic nerve health. Prevention, and especially non-toxic preventive approaches to therapy are critically important for anyone at risk, as well as those already showing damage. At best, conventional medical and surgical interventions attempt to check the advance of this progressive degenerative condition, but in many cases, blindness still is the final result. The following complementary modalities are worthy of consideration by the doctor and patient seeking the best long-term outcome.

Lifestyle, Stress Management & Exercise

Stress management and exercise

Socrates said, "Just as we cannot treat the eye without the head, and we cannot treat the head without the body, so we cannot treat the body without the soul."

Stress causes dilation of the pupil, which can increase IOP. Stress has long been known as one of the triggers of acute angle closure glaucoma attacks. As early as 1818, anxiety was linked to glaucoma attacks. Other risk factors, which interact with stress include narrow drainage angles in the eyes and anatomically short eyes. Holding feelings of resentment, anger and frustration seem to contribute to such an eye structure, especially during the formative childhood years. Stress also causes an immediate rise in IOP in glaucoma patients, while chronic stress eventually leads to increased eye pressure for anyone. Above average stress increases risk of ocular hypertension by 2.8 times. One study found that 100% of glaucoma patients experienced frustrating life experiences at the time their glaucoma began. Associated emotions ranged from anxiety to anger to depression, and during periods when patients' sense of security was most threatened, IOP and glaucoma symptoms were found to increase. Anxiety not only affects blood pressure, which is associated with glaucoma, but also increases the tendency of the blood to clot and triggers vasospasms in the retinal arteries. Many glaucoma patients show additional signs of stress including problems with sleep, digestion and loss of appetite. The glaucoma-prone individual tends to have a personality, which includes anxiety, perfectionism, nervousness, and hypersensitivity. An association between low levels of alcohol use and reduced ocular hypertension may be due either to reduced chronicity of stress patterns or simply to the cardiovascular benefits which are at least partially due the bioflavonoid content in red wine. Stress reduction through biofeedback of the frontalis muscle can also be helpful in lowering IOP. The simple act of relaxing and smiling, however, if achievable, results in essentially the same changes. IOP is never elevated when one is happy and tranquil. Biofeedback to increase skin temperature as a measure of the quality of circulation and smooth muscle relaxation is helpful in migraine and Raynaud's syndrome, both of which are related to glaucoma.

Whole body aerobic exercise has been shown to reduce IOP significantly, by 4.6 mm Hg, in previously sedentary glaucoma patients, with the most sedentary patients experiencing the greatest benefit. Even a single session of exercise such as 6 deep knee bends reduces IOP, and benefits continue for 3 weeks if exercise is discontinued. The amount of IOP reduction is as great as (and additive to) that obtained by using beta blocker eye drops, with increased pressure reductions achieved by more intense exercise. In normal and low-tension glaucoma, increased arterial partial pressure of carbon dioxide (pCO2), as produced by exercise, dilates blood vessels, increasing blood flow as well.

Normally, 30% of retinal ganglion cells die in 10 weeks of glaucoma caused by surgically blocking veinous drainage from the eye. After preconditioning with repeated periods of hypoxia, this was reduced to 3%, with neuroprotective effects lasting for months. Aerobic exercise to tolerance, that is getting a little out of breath, will produce this kind of intermittent hypoxia.

An optimal activity program might include 45 minutes of essentially non-stop physical activity such as walking, swimming, cycling or rebounding every other day, while others have recommended 10 to 30 minutes daily. One study found that 40 minutes of brisk walking 4 times a week for 3 months significantly reduced IOP. Interestingly, the seasonal variation in IOP is typically highest in the winter and lowest in the summer. Perhaps this is due to increase physical activity in the summer. The daily variation of IOP is also usually highest on waking, and has already decreased, even to normal levels, perhaps through lymph drainage due to physical activity, by the time it is measured in an eye doctor's office. The best exercise program for circulation and lymph drainage for the entire body, including the eyes is rebounding, with 12 minutes a day giving equivalent exercise to 40 minutes of jogging, yet without straining joints in the knees or low-back. On the other hand, jarring exercise may contribute to increased release of pigment in a specific condition known as pigmentary glaucoma. Pigmentary glaucoma tends to affect highly nearsighted individuals with dark pigmentation. Also, inverted postures, such as headstands, can increase IOP dramatically, reaching levels above 30 mm Hg in normals and even higher in those with glaucoma. In a few glaucoma suspects pressure even increases simply by lying down. When exercising, keep in mind that electrolytes such as zinc, potassium and magnesium are lost in sweating, so replacement of these minerals is important. Vision training, involving activities, which support enhanced efficiency and ease of eye movement have been shown in an unpublished study to reduce IOP. Looking to the side (lateral gaze) temporarily increases IOP by about 2 or 3 mm Hg. More frequent eye movements into lateral gaze may function to pump fluid out of the eye more efficiently, similar to the pumping of lymph through general body movements, resulting in a long-term decrease in IOP. Eye movement in general tends to increase with increased gross motor activity. Both glaucoma and myopia, which seem to be closely related in their pathophysiology, appear to involve a lack of eye movement. In myopia, eye movement is greater when wearing contact lenses compared to glasses, but contacts should not be worn overnight, since this can affect eye-pressure. Daily-massage of the eyes and orbit can help achieve a lower pressure in the eye by improving drainage of aqueous humor, lymph and venous blood. "Eye Points" is a recommended massage program that includes not only the bony orbit, but also body accupressure points that trigger improved drainage in the eye area. These relaxation techniques as well as "Palming should be used during frequent breaks in any visually centered task such as reading, computer work, or watching television. Eye Stretch is a recommended exercise to improve lymphatic and veinous drainage for the eye area while releasing tension in the extra-ocular muscle system. Performance lenses or other plus lenses for closework have been shown to help reduce IOP by reducing the demand for contraction of the ciliary muscle which controls eye focus. Quitting smoking is critically important, since by itself, nicotine can raise IOP. One herbal program has been proven 99% effective for quitting smoking within 7 days. Avoiding any other toxic drugs and food additives, as much as possible is also paramount, as many of these may have a similar effect. Detoxification is very important in the long run to remove the accumulated toxins in the body, but this should proceed gently so as not to trigger increased pressure during healing crises. Avoiding toxins in the diet, such as pesticides, is important, too. Peel commercially grown fruit, and wash vegetables before cooking. Steaming vegetables lightly also helps to remove volatile pesticide. Weight loss and natural reduction of hypertension are helpful, too. Both of these factors, along with myopia, are associated with ocular hypertension. Pharmacological reduction of high blood pressure in the presence of ocular hypertension can actually increase glaucomatous damage to the optic nerve due to the creation of an increased pressure differential at the optic nerve head, increasing cupping and reducing capillary perfusion to the nerve fibers. Even clothing can affect IOP and visual fields. Neckties can increase IOP by compressing the jugular veins, reducing veinous drainage from the head and eye area. In one study, 67% of businessmen in normal health wore neckties tight enough to reduce visual performance. None of us, especially someone with glaucoma or at risk of it, needs this kind of added stress, so loosen up those neckties just a notch, and now you're dressed for success. Like a famous boxer used to say, "Float like a butterfly, sting like a bee, your hands can't hit what your eyes don't see." And then there's also the old addage, "use it or lose it." This certainly applies to the use of our peripheral vision and related eye and body movement in maintaining our spatial vision, whether in glaucoma, or under any kind of stress conditions.

Mileau: Water & Biological Terrain

Water & Biological Terrain

In most cases, glaucoma is a chronic degenerative condition, resulting from Phase 1 conditions in the brain, eye and optic nerve area. This is also the terrain for viral conditions, and an association is seen with 28% of patients who have herpes eye infections experiencing secondary glaucoma. Phase 1 terrain is excessively oxidized, resulting in oxidation of circulating LDL cholesterol, which deposits and hardens on the inner lining of the blood vessels, impairing their ability to dilate normally, thus restricting circulation. The retina of the eye has the highest oxygen demand of any tissue in the body, with local hypoxia or ischemia in the nerve fibers of the retina and optic nerve leading to further free radical activity. Lipid peroxidation can be especially destructive in the optic nerve area with its myelinated nerve fibers containing a high concentration of fatty acids, which can produce a chain reaction of reactive oxygen species. It is also known that lipid peroxidation occurs in the degeneration of cells in the anterior chamber angle that drains the fluid from the eye.

Phase 1 terrain is also characterized by excessive alkalinity in the veinous blood. This is primarily due to a blocked and inefficient cellular energy metabolism, resulting in lack of acid metabolic wastes such as carbonic acid. Steroid eye drops, for example, induce a Phase

1 terrain in the eye. It has been shown that they alkalize the aqueous humor in proportion to the rise in IOP, while at the same time depleting antioxidant defenses. Vitamin C levels fall by 50 to 80% throughout the eye. Thus circulation, oxygenation and cellular respiration in addition to antioxidant protection (especially the fat soluble antioxidants) are critical components to provide the physiological system if it is to mount a successful remission from this Phase 1 terrain.

Drinking a lot of fluids all at once can temporarily raise IOP as much as 30%. This does not mean glaucoma patients should drink less water. As with all medicines, though, the source, energy, purity, contents, dosage and frequency are all crucial. All water is not the same. Water with anything added, such as tea, coffee, soda, or juice reduces the water's ability to carry nutrients and toxins in the body, as its solvent ability is already in use.

Diuretic effects of caffeine and alcohol

When caffeine or alcohol among the contents, drinking actually depletes your body's water stores, since these chemicals act as diuretics. Dehydrated cells are thirsty for more fluid to improve their health and function, so you will want to drink more beer or soda, making matters even worse, except for the corporate stock holders. In glaucoma, your ciliary body may be getting the message from your eye tissues that more fluid is needed because of intracellular dehydration. Medications may try to block this response, but do not supply the water your cells need!

Acid waters

Most waters are also oxidizing agents, using up antioxidants and promoting free radical damage of tissues such as the optic nerve in glaucoma. Tap water is the worst in this category as it typically contains added chlorine. Most waters are acidic, adding to the toxic burden on the kidneys and pushing tissues toward inflammation, which is counterproductive in glaucoma. Soda is the worst in this aspect, with added carbonation (CO_2), a metabolic waste product, which forms carbonic acid, and phosphoric acid, which is even more acidic. Most bottled waters are intentionally acidified to help prevent living organisms from flourishing. Drinking anything over about 4 ounces of any of the conventional types of water, including tap water, bottled water, or RO or other filtered water, at one time. Drinking 4 ounces of good pure water every half hour on the other hand, increases lymph flow and detoxification. After a few days of regularity with a balanced water regimen, the kidneys are able to improve their eliminative function, which is foundational to support healing of many underlying causes of glaucoma, whether open or narrow angle.

Where acid water does make sense is topically, on the skin. The skin naturally tries to maintain an acid mantle and a layer of oil to inhibit growth of pathogens and maintain the skin's important barrier function. Soaps destroy these purposeful protective mechanisms by alkalizing and removing oils. Acid microwater is a better solvent than other waters for cleansing the skin, and works without disrupting the barrier function. A stronger version made in special units requiring addition of specific minerals to support a stronger ionization, called superoxide water, is used in place of all topical antibiotics in those Japanese hospitals that utilize the technology. This astringent healing water is so potent that it can prevent the need for amputation in cases of gangrene.

Microwater

Far better is microwater, which has water clusters about half the size of filtered water. This allows microwater to penetrate 10 times better not only into the blood, but into the extracellular fluid, the lymph and the intracellular space where it is actually needed, carrying essential nutrients in, and acids, wastes and toxins out. Because microwater units produce two streams of water, alkaline and acid, alkaline minerals are concentrated in the water used internally for drinking and cooking. This extra alkalinity is helpful to counterbalance the acidity produced by stress, inefficient metabolism in toxic, damaged tissues, and the highly acidifying Standard American Diet (SAD) rich in sugar, refined carbohydrate, grains and heavily cooked commercial meats, as well as pharmaceuticals. Because of the enhanced penetrating effect of microwater, it helps digest food, even when taken at mealtime, and does not excessively dilute the blood, so it doesn't strain the kidneys to maintain blood homeostasis. Microwater is also directly antioxidant, as it carries a negative electrical potential, measured in millivolts as rH2 (Hydrogen Potential) or ORP (Oxidation Reduction Potential). This means that this highly penetrating water, made of molecules about 10 times smaller than Vitamin C, which is the smallest of the conventionally considered nutritional antioxidants, and even over 3 times smaller than urea, one of the most potent antioxidants in the body. Even the entire micro-structured water cluster is smaller than TMG, the smallest anti-oxidant in the diet.

Hypertension and ocular hypertension are linked, and both may be significantly related to chronic dehydration. Chronic dehydration, resulting in increased blood viscosity, can be caused by diuretics or simply by the Standard American Diet (SAD), which includes more soda than water. Increased IOP has also been associated with constipation, which is closely linked to fluid metabolism. After about 3 days of regular consumption of water, the kidneys are able to readapt and increase the efficiency of their filtration of the blood as well. The best water is that which is filtered to remove unwanted chemicals, such as heavy metals, chlorine, fluoride and pesticide residues, and then ionized. Bioelectronics of Vincent (BEV) quality filtration can be achieved by a multi-stage filter system incorporating reverse osmosis with other water purification technologies. Ionization by electrolysis imparts a negative charge, which provides the most effective biocompatible anti-oxidant known. It also restructures the water, reducing the average molecular cluster size from about 16 to about 8 water molecules according to NMR studies, resulting in a 10-fold increase in penetration into the lymphatic system and even the intracellular spaces. This water, a better solvent than tap water, increases nutrient absorption and utilization, while also enhancing elimination of metabolic wastes and other toxins from tissue stores. The alkaline-reduced water that is used for drinking and cooking accelerates the body's healing process, which initially involves the re-establishment of efficient mitochondrial aerobic metabolism followed by the shift from Phase 1 to Phase 2 terrain. This water releases oxygen specifically to those tissues, which are eliminating toxins, including the toxins, which are released in unblocking mitochondrial electron transport chain enzymes. (see also: Feldman RM, Steinmann WC, Spaeth GL et al: Effects of altered daily fluid intake on intraocular pressure in glaucoma patients. Glaucoma 1987; 9: 118-121.)

Osmotic agents like vitamin C, glycerine and salt decrease IOP by pulling fluid from the eyes. They also increase biological energy (measured in microwatts) in the blood, shifting terrain away from Phase 1, which is the low energy zone in which medically treated glaucoma is most prevalent.

High body temperature, characteristic of Phase 2 terrain (e.g. associated with bacterial infection, healing crisis and spontaneous remission), is related to a temporary increase in IOP. This can, however, if not suppressed by antibiotics or antipyretics like aspirin, lead to resolution of the internal causes of the problem, followed by remission from the disease. If there is damage to the myelin sheath of the optic nerve fibers, as in MS, increased body temperature from exercise or a hot bath can temporarily worsen visual fields.

When complementary medicine is used early in the natural history of glaucoma, or in later stages to attempt a more intensive approach to reversal and rehabilitation of eye health and function, the body's direct attempts to heal underlying causes such as allergy and toxicity are almost certain to surface, as supportive vital functions such as more robust circulation and vigorous immune system responses are restored. These are reflected in a Phase 4, Cleansing terrain, characterized by hyper physiological responses, which are particularly challenging to manage as an inter-current therapy while still on a course of standard suppressive glaucoma medications. This is work that should ideally be taken on by an experienced holistic eye doctor or a seasoned team with good communication.

In the case where effective movement toward resolution of underlying causes is achieved, it is likely that serial oscillations will be required between Phase 4, Cleansing, and Phase 3, Regeneration, as clearing of toxins, immune complexes, stored excess protein and cellular debris makes way for regeneration of functional parenchymal cells. Phase 5, Balancing issues dealing with life stresses and hormonal regulation will typically emerge at later stages of the retracing as earlier, deeper causal factors are unraveled through the well-selected application of complementary medicine modalities and remedies.

Many glaucoma patients are using complementary medicine. (Rhee DJ, Spaeth GL, Terebuh A, Myers JS, Augsburger JJ, Shatz L, Ritner JA, Katz LJ. Prevalence of the use of complementary & alternative medicine (CAM) for glaucoma. Ophthalmology 2002; 109: 438-443.)

CSF and the optic nerve

While IOP is easy to measure clinically, the aqueous humor is not actually the fluid that nourishes the optic nerve head where damage is seen in glaucoma. The flow of extracellular fluids in the eye is normally from the Cerebrospinal Fluid (CSF) through the optic nerve head and forward through the vitreous and lens into the aqueous, which drains out the front of the eye into the veins and lymph. While glaucoma is sometimes associated with elevated IOP, normal tension glaucoma is associated with reduced CSF pressure, so in either case an elevated backwards pressure at the optic nerve head may be a common causal feature of the glaucomas.

CSF is produced by the choroid plexus, and within each diurnal cycle the total volume is reabsorbed into the cranial circulation in the superior sagittal sinus through arachnoid villi. A recent study has shown that CNS neurons shrink during sleep widening the intercellular space between cells. This allows flow of CSF, which flushes out accumulated wastes including amyloid that accumulates in neurodegenerative conditions including glaucoma. This newly documented CSF flow into brain tissue is through spaces on the outside of blood vessels and between glial cells. The space between glial cells increased by 60% with unconsciosness whether from sleep, anesthesia, or induced by blocking norepinephrine, which regulates cell volume. The change in intercellular space made a dramatic difference in the flow of CSF and clearance of dyes and large molecules. Radiolabeled beta-amyloid cleared faster during the sleep mode.

(Xie et al "Sleep initiated fluid flux drives metabolite clearance from the adult brain." Science, October 18, 2013. DOI:: 10.1126/science.1241224)

(Research published summer 2012 in Science Translational Medicine by Dr. Maiken Nedergaard at the University of Rochester Medical Center in New York using 2 photon microscopy on living tissue, with follow-on studies underway at OHSU.)

http://ninds.nih.gov/news_and_events/news_articles/pressrelease_br ain_sleep_10182013.htm

The subarachnoid space around the optic nerve is filled with CSF, though not normally macroscopically filled with CSF, unless the intracranial pressure is elevated. Papilledema manifests and recent evidence of chemistry gradients between the bulk CSF and that around the optic nerve supports the idea that under such conditions, the optic nerve area effectively becomes a separate fluid compartment isolated from full communication with the bulk of the CSF.

Healing Glaucoma

Grossly, it is a potential space that is continuous with the rest of the subarachnoid space surrounding the brain, which is filled with CSF, so whatever extracellular fluid does surround the optic nerve is part of the CSF compartment. The same is true for the extracellular fluid between nerve fibers in the optic nerve, which is technically not a nerve, but a tract of the central nervous system by its embryological origin.

There is also centrifugal flow of CSF through the optic nerve cul de sac. India ink injected in the SAS of the optic nerve drains into the dural lymphatics. (Killer, et al. 1999) Together with the new evidence of a diurnal glial pump mechanism surrounding the vasculature, there appears to be primarily a central to peripheral flow of CSF around and within the optic nerve that becomes congested and stagnant in papilledema. Contrast dye in the CSF does not show up in the optic nerve compartment under these conditions. This could explain why some patients sustain papilledema and vision loss despite having a CSF lumboperitoneal shunt to relieve intracranial pressure (Kelman, et al. 1991)

A lesser degree of CSF congestion at the optic nerve head likely exists in some glaucomas, such as atypical normotensive glaucoma. In glaucomatous optic neuropathy, astrocytes are activated, and levels of matrix metallo-proteinases, tumor necrosis factor alpha and endothelin increase. These factors can cause arachnoiditis, reducing CSF inflow, and can also contribute to optic nerve damage.

Endothelin levels are increased systemically in glaucoma, reducing both microcirculation and axoplasmic transport (Hernandez, 2000).

Studies of anterior optic neuritis shows that inflammation can precede sheath and disc swelling, so inflammatory processes are likely involved early in the causal chain that blocks optic nerve CSF outflow. On autopsy, polymorphonuclear leucocytes are found attached to the arachnoid, even in people with no neurological diagnoses (Killer, 2003a). With introduction of a foreign bacterium, additional immune cells seen included macrophages, lymphoblasts and monocytes (Merchant and Low, 1977). Inflammatory responses, even to subarachnoid hemorrhage, can produce fibrotic micro-scarring secondary to arachnoiditis and trabeculitis, inhibiting outflow including by closing the arachnoid apertures that drain into the meningeal lymphatics, and promoting ischemia.

Increased levels of L-PGDS (Lipocalin-like Prostaglandin D-Synthase) in the CSF during local congestion increases neuroprotection for astrocytes, increases apoptosis, and modulates inflammatory processes. The optic nerve head is the most sequestered from the general CSF flow and would therefore be the most at risk. This is also a site where myelination of nerve fibers ends, and unmyelinated fibers containing a much higher concentration of mitochondria begins, again making this an area especially vulnerable to hypoxia and ischemia. Damage to the microvasculature in the supportive septa of pia matter and to the mitochondria they serve is likely related to vision loss, i.e. loss of function of the optic nerve axons, as demonstrated in the extreme in Leber's hereditary optic neuropathy (Biousse and Newman, 2001).

CSF pressure (normally 11-13 mm Hg) is elevated in Ocular Hypertension (usually 12-13 mm Hg), but reduced (usually 8-10 mm Hg) in Primary Open Angle Glaucoma, and reduced even more in Normal Tension Glaucoma (p=.013). Amazingly, neurons can resist uniform pressures of 3800 mm Hg, but pressure gradients of only 3-4 mm Hg, such as the translaminar pressure difference at the optic nerve head traversing the lamina cribrosa can stop axoplasmic transport, which can cause cell death. This explains why Normal Tension Glaucoma outcomes improve dramatically when IOPs are reduced to 11 mm Hg.

The lamina is normally 457 microns thick but thins to 201 microns in glaucoma, further accentuating the gradient. Translaminar pressure differences are normally less than 3 mm Hg, but run 3 to 20 mm Hg in glaucoma, including Normal Tension Glaucoma. Normally the IOP and CSF pressure are very highly correlated (p<.001) and related to blood pressure (p<.04), since both fluids are produced from the blood. When IOP and CSF pressures are measured on the same day, the translaminar pressure gradient is significantly (p < .001) correlated with visual field loss (correlation coefficient .69), while IOP and CSF pressure do not independently show significant correlation in multivariate analysis.

The fluid metabolism is disturbed in glaucoma. Normally there is significant correlation between blood pressure and CSF pressure (correlation coefficient .24) and close coordination between CSF pressure and IOP (correlation coefficient .76, p<.001). In ocular hypertension, CSF pressure is elevated. Even in acutely elevated CSF pressure, there is some mixed evidence of correlation with IOP. This functional coherence is disrupted in the low CSF pressure of glaucoma, a type of compartment syndrome where biocommunication based coordination of functions is lost. This is consistent with blocked regulation and a Phase 1 terrain in a chronic degenerative condition.

The body's innate healing processes that could potentially restore a healthy pattern of function would be expected to potentially produce a healing crisis with not only elevated IOP but simultaneously elevated (and protective) CSF pressure. Since CSF pressure is difficult and invasive to measure, it is a challenge to discern between such a healing crisis and a disease crisis, so in standard practice all acute reactive phases are suppressed if possible. Thus spontaneous remission under medical treatment is not observed even if it may be possible. It is analogous to cancer in which if every bacterial infection and high fever were effectively suppressed by antibiotics, we would see no spontaneous remission at all.

In Normal Tension Glaucoma, systemic blood pressure is often low (possible blocked regulation) and there is a pattern of vasospasms (negative regulation), both of which may contribute to loss of perfusion and ischemia of the optic nerve head, but do not account for the morphological changes around the optic nerve head which are like those in high tension Primary Open Angle Glaucoma. Characteristic changes include increased cupping related to a bulging out posteriorly of the lamina cribrosa, loss of neuroretinal rim tissue and expansion of the area of parapapillary atrophy. Optic neuropathies due to vascular issues (other than Arteritic Anterior Ischemic Optic Neuropathy) generally do not cause these changes.

CSF has lower than normal protein level in glaucoma. This may reflect a deficiency in clearing of waste proteins such as amyloid that build up in neurodegenerative conditions.

Diet, Food Sensitivities and Allergies

A study of 113 patients with chronic simple glaucoma showed immediate IOP increases of up to 20 mm Hg upon challenge (exposure) with food or other allergens. Another study of 3 individual cases of simple glaucoma showed that elimination of food allergens markedly improved treatment outcomes compared to treatment with drugs and surgery or drugs alone. In one case, intraocular pressure could only be controlled once allergens were eliminated from the diet. In two other cases, despite adequate control of IOP with a combination of drugs and surgery, visual field loss continued to progress. Visual fields actually improved markedly upon beginning an allergen-free diet. This illustrates an important factor in glaucoma, that it is not simply a matter of pressure, but rather a complex interaction of biophysical and biochemical parameters that influence the cellular metabolism and function in the retinal ganglion cells and their axons in the optic nerve. Allergy responses are known to cause altered vascular permeability and vasospasm, which could result in the congestion and edema found in glaucoma. Sjogren first identified the relationship between allergy and IOP. As early as 1947, research showed that uncontrollable cases of glaucoma resolved on an allergy-free diet. Antihistamine treatment has proven effective in glaucoma patients with allergies, after conventional treatment failed. Glaucoma in just one eye has even been found to be frequently due to sleeping with that eye against a feather pillow. In the trabecular meshwork, histamine increases intracellular influx of calcium, increasing smooth muscle tension and potentially reducing circulation. Histamine has been shown to cause a reduction in the ability of the trabecular meshwork cells to keep the meshwork clear of debris, resulting in increased intraocular pressure. Antigen studies now also show a link to autoimmune processes. Until individual testing of food reactions can be performed, many practitioners recommend as a minimum beginning with elimination of tobacco, sugar, coffee and tea (including decaf; herb teas are allowed), alcohol, white flour and other refined and processed foods, with reduction of commercially raised dairy products and red meats. Any beverages, preferably microwater (which can pass through the eye more readily), should be taken evenly throughout the day rather than drinking a lot at one time, which can raise IOP. Airborne allergens should be eliminated through the use of ozone, oxozone, or HEPA filtration units, although oxozone appears to be the most efficient method. MSG may be a significant trigger of glaucoma, too. Glutamate has been found at elevated levels in the vitreous of glaucoma patients. Glutamate is known to be toxic to retinal ganglion cells and is known to cause circulatory disturbances such as vasospasms. Glutamate is an excitatory amino acid linked to neurological diseases such as Parkinson's and Alzheimer's. Acetyl-L-Carnitine, glutathione, vitamin B3, and CoQ10 are neuroprotective by preventing depletion of ATP, since it is in low energy states (Phase 1) that nerve cells are damaged by glutamate. It has been suggested to reduce commercial meats, dairy, salt and nuts, while including lots of vegetables along with cold-water fish and eggs from free-ranging chickens. Moderate egg consumption may increase beneficial HDL without significant increase of LDL. One study using a low fat diet centered on rice and vegetables together with nutritional supplements achieved rapid (within 2 days) and sustained reduction in IOP of 5 to 7 mm Hg, which is better than results with current medical therapies. This study was done at Duke University in 1949! Five servings of fresh organic produce (fruits and vegetables) per day are recommended. Green leafy vegetables, such as collards, kale, mustard greens and spinach are suggested as a source of xanthophyll carotenoids, which help protect the optic nerve fibers, especially in the central vision area. Buckwheat is beneficial due to its high content of the bioflavonoid rutin.

Neuroprotection

Glaucoma is the diagnosis, a name or label for the damage that impairs our vision, but the damage itself occurs by specific chemical pathways. While there are probably thousands of different triggers, including many different neurotoxins, like pesticides and heavy metals, they all have some things in common that makes it easier to deal with when it comes to prevention and healing.

Causal pathways converge on key deficiency states like oxidation (electron deficiency), which is contributed to by hypoxia (oxygen deficiency), which is exacerbated by acidity (alkaline macromineral deficiency). The alkaline minerals are used up over time to buffer the acid effects of environmental toxins, pharmaceuticals, endotoxins produced in the gut, and excitotoxins resulting from stress and the modern diet. In an acid state, oxygen becomes bound and unavailable. That is why fish die from acid rain. Our cells are like the fish, their lake is the extracellular fluid, and modern life supplies the acidity in all the forms just listed. Without oxygen, the nerve cells lose 95% of their energy. They may be alive, but they can no longer function to support vision. They are blind. All the retinal cells may be on the edge of this condition, especially since the retina is the highest oxygen demanding tissue in the body.

The first cells to lose function are usually in Bjerrum's area since the circulation to these cells is the most easily stressed at the optic nerve head, where cross-linking of collagen fibers constricts blood perfusion of the local microcirculation. This causes ischemia (circulation deficiency), which feeds both the oxygen deficiency (hypoxia) and acidity (buffer deficiency), since inefficient (anaerobic) metabolism leaves a residual sludge of lactic acid that builds up in the cells and causes them to swell. The swelling of acidic tissue further contributes to ischemia. At this point the cause and effect can go round and round, resulting in a chronic state of ill health in the affected optic nerve fiber areas. This intracellular swelling and inflammation (extracellular swelling) also associated with an increase in acidity (excess protons is another way to describe this state) ties up not only the oxygen now needed more than ever to finish burning up the waste lactic acid into carbon dioxide (gas) and water, but ties up more and more water, both in the lactic acid itself, and by binding water osmotically, to keep the acid wastes from being too concentrated, toxic and irritating. This is a state of dehydration, which makes it harder for the needed water and alkaline minerals and oxygen to penetrate into the area. The dehydration also contributes to further connective tissue damage with deposition of dehydrated sheets of proteins called amyloid associated with glaucoma as with other neurodegenerative conditions.

Typically the difference between various diseases is not so much in the nature of the pathophysiology, but primarily in the location of the

52

process. The typical culprits, almost always involved in some way in each human being's natural history of attempted self-healing includes fundamental and common insults like psychoemotional stress, environmental toxicity, endotoxicity, acidity, trauma, allergy, and inflammation.

Here we will focus on some major final common pathways of tissue damage that all of those intermediate causes trigger. We ultimately need to address the original and intermediate causes whenever possible to eliminate the tendency toward damage and degeneration by accelerating the body's completion of healing processes related to past insults. While those causes or at least residues are being identified and eliminated over time, according to the body's sequence of healing which is typically in the reverse order in which they were accumulated (retracing), we need to consider how to mitigate the tissue damage at its simpler common endpoints of oxidation (electron deficiency), glycation (sugar deposition) and other toxic deposition.

Connective tissue damage and shrinkage due to crosslinking (dehydration and micro-scarring by disulfide (sulfur to sulfur) bridges between proteins. In amyloid protein deposits, which are strongly associated with glaucoma and other neurodegenerative disease processes, two layers of beta-sheet protein deposits interdigitate to create compact dehydrated interface termed as steric-zipper interface.

Neurotoxins

Neurotoxins involved in glaucoma include excitotoxins, heavy metals, pesticides, PCBs and other environmental toxins, as well as endotoxins produced in the body, such as methyl mercury and mercuric chloride made 1000 times more toxic (to create a zone of immunosuppression) by dysbiotic bacteria and fungi from metallic mercury, and indol and scatol made by putrefaction of undigested proteins by dysbiotic gut flora.   The full solution for healing these underlying causes of glaucoma involves both neuroprotection and removal of the toxins that damage the nerve cells.   Neuroprotection is offered by increasing levels of antioxidants, anti-glycation agents and other remedies that help with the five phases of healing according to a model I developed based on the observations of European Biological Medicine and Bioelectronics of Vincent measurements of the biophysical terrain in people while they were progressing into deeper phases of disease, and then while they were reversing and retracing those same steps and moving through the same terrains defined by measurements of the concentrations of the most basic particles of physics that define our health: protons (pH), electrons (rH2 or ORP) and photons (ionization measured by resistivity or impedence).   Together, these are the parameters that define biological energy in microwatts according to the Nernst equation in physics.

Phase 1 involves cellular detoxification of heavy metals, pesticides, PCBs and any other key neurotoxins blocking intracellular metabolic pathways including aerobic metabolism and epigenetic regulation of the DNA, leading to the ability to stimulate regeneration of the mitochondria for increased cellular energy production and cellular function, such as restoration of visual field areas where cells are not dead but just not functional. This phase is crucial whenever there are viruses, low-grade fevers or any chronic degenerative disease issues.

Phase 2 is typically seen as a rapid phase of cellular repair and rejuvenation of metabolic enzyme functions including the anti-oxidant enzyme system. This phase also deals with issues of bacterial dysbiosis, bacterial infection, high fevers and parasites.

Phase 3 involves tissue regeneration, as well as clearing the way for this restoration of normal healthy tissue by eliminating any dead tissue and the fungi that feed on that dead matter.

Phase 4 connective tissue detoxification as well as immune modulation for reduction of inflammation, allergy and autoimmune responses.

Phase 5 deals with balancing of endocrine and life stress factors to reduce cortisol and excitotoxin production. Personal and spiritual growth are central to this process.

The specific sequence of phases and the systems, organs and tissues that require healing are unique to each person. The amount of time it takes to clear detoxification issues, whether it is intracellular in Phase 1 or extracellular in Phase 4 depends upon the location and identity of the toxins, as well as the gross quantity of each toxin and the degree of functionality in the relevant elimination systems, as well as how well the remedy support program is tailored to the unique needs of the individual in real time. This is where methods of biocommunication become essential to fine-tune the healing support program in real time, at least on a monthly cycle during intensive health restoration.

Accelerated self-healing can be a bit like a roller coaster ride, as the body can go through flu-like detoxification or cleansing reactions, also referred to as healing crises, particularly in Phase 2. Optimum results are obtainable when we can be guided through these retracings and Herxheimer, or die-off reactions gently with a minimum of suppressive medications such as antipyretics, synthetic antibiotics (fungal toxin analogs and sulfa drugs), steroid medications, anti-inflammatory drugs and pain killers. Increased intake of drainage remedies and neuroprotective remedies, temporary reduction or cessation of intake of detoxification remedies, and emphasis on microwater intake, positive healing intention and rest is usually sufficient, along with the knowledge that the symptoms represent a healing crisis, the body's focused, intelligent action to restore health.

There are key differences between a healing crisis and a disease crisis that help to distinguish the two. In a healing crisis, elimination systems such as the bowels, urination and sweating are working well or even beyond their usual capacity. This can be further facilitated with enemas or colonics, drinking microwater and taking Far Infrared saunas. Rest and sleep tend to be more than usual in a healing crisis, though discomfort may be a challenge, while they may be very disturbed or absent in a disease crisis. Metabolism will be increased by fever in many healing crises.

For example, in over 2000 medically documented cases of spontaneous remission of cancer (a condition that occurs only in Phase 1, like most glaucomatous damage), every case showed Phase 2 indicators including a high fever and a bacterial infection. Bacteria cannot grow in Phase 1 terrain, so it is the body's healing of the conditions that allowed the bacteria to grow, producing enzymes that assisted in lysing (breaking down) the cancerous tumors within a few days in every case. In any case, whether flu-like symptoms represent a worsening of health or a healing reaction, an updated assessment of the body's needs during any health crisis is essential for optimal accelerated self-healing.

Once any needed healing crises are past and basic cellular physiology is restored, there is often a need to cycle through multiple phases of tissue cleansing and regeneration, and all phases may need to be repeated as the body gets strong enough to cleanse and repair various damaged organs and systems, especially the eliminative organs that filter the blood, the liver and kidneys, because of the toxic age in which we live. Both are extremely relevant in glaucoma, and the kidneys are particularly challenging because, like the eye, they are wrapped tightly in connective tissue (the sclera in the case of the eye). This means that both the kidneys and the eyes may prefer a moderately slow pace of accelerated self-healing, not a pushy chemical approach with heavy doses of drugs, herbs or even megavitamins. Gentle, soothing but deeply effective therapies like Far Infrared saunas, microwater, Syntonic phototherapy, flower essences and homeopathy are perfect to emphasize.

Excitotoxicity

Excess of excitatory neurotransmitters Glutamate (as contained in Mono Sodium Glutamate) and N-Methyl-D-aspartate (NMDA), an amino acid derivative, which acts as a specific agonist at the NMDA receptor appear to contribute to nerve cell death in glaucoma. Intracellular deposits of mishandled Calcium in glaucoma are a typical effect of this excitotoxicity.

Avoiding Aspartame, as well as MSG, including all of its hidden dietary forms, is a good initial step in reducing this risk factor.

Aspartame

Aspartame is a dipeptide made of Aspartic acid and Phenylalanine. In the presence of moisture, it breaks down at room temperature to produce methanol, also know as wood alcohol, which is famous for causing blindness. More symptom complaints are reported to the FDA from Aspartame than any other regulated chemical today.

MSG

Mono Sodium Glutamate (MSG) was originally discovered in seaweeds that can carry a very high content, so watch the oriental snacks like o-senbei, arare and seaweeds if you want to heal your glaucoma. MSG is also frequently masked on product labels under a variety of names. These ingredients always contain the amino acid Glutamate or Glutamic Acid:

Glutamic acid (European food additive identifier: E 620), Glutamate (E 620),

Monosodium glutamate (E 621) or Natrium glutamate

Monopotassium glutamate (E 622)

Calcium glutamate (E 623)

Monoammonium glutamate (E 624)

Magnesium glutamate (E 625)

Anything "hydrolyzed", any "hydrolyzed protein" (except hydrolyzed rice or whey proteins for supporting protein sparing fasting as part of a meal substitute plan)

Calcium caseinate, Sodium caseinate

Yeast food, yeast nutrient, yeast extract, autolyzed yeast

Ajinomoto, Ac'cent, Vetsin (trade names for MSG)

Gelatin

Textured protein, or any "…protein"

Soy protein, soy protein concentrate, soy protein isolate

Whey protein, whey protein concentrate, whey protein isolate

MSG is often also found or produced by these food ingredients:

Carrageenan (E 407)

Bouillon and broth

Stock

Any "flavors" or "flavoring"

Maltodextrin

Citric acid, Citrate (E 330)

Anything "ultra-pasteurized"

Barley malt

Pectin (E 440)

Anything "enzyme modified" or containing "enzymes" or protease

Malt extract

Soy sauce or soy sauce extract

Anything "protein fortified"

Anything "fermented"

Seasonings

The following foods can also trigger excitotoxin (MSG) reactions in sensitive people, and are thus best avoided by those with glaucoma:

Corn starch

Corn syrup

Modified food starch

Lipolyzed butter fat

Dextrose

Rice syrup and brown rice syrup

Milk powder

Reduced fat milk including skim milk, 1% milk and 2% milk

Low fat and fat-free foods

Enriched and vitamin enriched foods

This doesn't mean you can't or shouldn't eat any protein, because everyone needs protein, but you do want to minimize the total amount of glutamine in your diet, so emphasize high quality, digestible or pre-digested protein, and skip the rest.

Excess & Indigestible Protein

The thing to realize and change is that the Standard American Diet contains about four times too much protein. Excess protein becomes indigestible by exceeding our enzymatic digestive capacity. Poorly and partially digested protein may still be absorbed as larger particles and congest the lymphatic system, contributing to congestion of lymphatic drainage around the eyes, and therefore reduced outflow facility and increased IOP in glaucoma, as well as deposition of excess protein in the connective tissue of the extracellular spaces, on top of contributing to the excitotoxin deposition within the ganglion cells, causing vision loss in glaucoma.

Dehydrated Denatured Protein

One reason that a lot of protein we eat is not digestible is if it is cooked beyond rare in air, such as fried or baked, as this dehydrates the proteins, reducing the space available for enzymes to access the nitrogen bonds for hydrolysis in the digestive process. Think about how meat gets tougher as it is cooked to medium and well done, versus how stewed meats get more tender with cooking. Meat tenderizers can be helpful as they actually use proteolytic enzymes to tenderize, or partially pre-digest the proteins.

Excessively Large Protein Molecules

Another factor that adds to the protein problem is ingestion of excessively large protein molecules from soy, as well as gluten in wheat, and casein in cow milk and cow cheese. All three of these foods are among the top 7 food allergens, and this is one of the main reasons.

Putrefied Protein Toxins

Undigested protein provides food for pathogenic putrefactive bacteria in the gut, forming highly toxic amino acids that stress the kidneys and nerve cells like those in the retina that are energetically governed by the kidneys and the water element in the Oriental Medicine perspective. In the small intestine, the main toxin produced by this bacterial dysbiosis is indol, while in the large intestine it is scatol, also known as cadaverine because it is the putrid toxin that makes dead bodies smell so bad. So, if it stinks coming out, it wasn't properly digested, and has become a toxic load adding to the glaucoma problem. If the stool smells like something died, that is scatol. There is a simple in-office Indican test available to screen the urine for indole. Aside from cutting excess and indigestible protein from the diet, supplementing beneficial flora, digestive enzymes, herbal bitters that stimulate digestion, and a homeopathic digestive stimulant like my Digestzymes formula (from which I receive no royalty) are all worthy ideas to consider.

Microwaved Protein

A new addition to the protein problem is the use of microwaves in cooking, which break nitrogen bonds in the cooked proteins, making them indigestible to our proteolytic enzymes even if they are smaller or taken in appropriate quantities. When research subjects were fed only microwaved food, their live blood cells became indistinguishable from those of cancer patients (Phase 1, low energy terrain, where most degenerative glaucoma damage also occurs) within just 2 weeks.

Antioxidants

Oxidation is one of the key mechanisms by which our cells become damaged, whether by trauma, toxicity, aging, or the effects of disease processes in glaucoma. Oxidation means the loss of an electron. Oxidation is how fire burns wood into ash. Oxidation is promoted by free radicals, which are typically the result of high-energy electrons escaping the electron transport chain due to deficiency of cofactors like B Vitamins, Coenzyme Q10, or Oxygen, the ultimate receiver of spent electrons, in the mitochondria. The reactive compounds, often in the form of reactive oxygen species (ROS), carrying those electrons are looking to steal another electron to become stable. They are like a short circuit in the wiring of the cell's electrical system looking for a ground. And like a short circuit anywhere, they can do a lot of mischief, or even burn down the house. Anti-oxidants are our first line of defense against these ROS, since anti-oxidants by definition are electron donors.

So what can we do to protect our nerve cells and our vision, as we begin to unravel and repair this kind up accumulated damage and deposition? Let's look at the many antioxidants that, if they can penetrate into the area of damage, have the ability to donate an electron instead of having an electron stolen from some even more important part of the cell... In our tour of the many antioxidants in the retina and optic nerve, we will travel from the smallest, the humble electron itself, to the largest, our anti-oxidant enzymes:

Electrons (chemical symbol e-) have a molecular weight of zero (0) daltons. The top source is the earth, when the body is grounded to it. The second most abundant potential source is the air when we are around moving water and plants or a negative ion generator. Third is our drinking water when it is a pure mountain stream cascading over rocks in a pristine environment, or in today's real world, microwater. Fourth is our diet when it is obtained fresh from living plants and animals.

Water Molecules (chemical formula: $H_2 O$) have a molecular weight of 18 daltons. Most water is depleted in electrons by adding chlorine, processing and running through metal pipes, making it an oxidizing agent, promoting further free radical damage in glaucoma.

Urea ($C_1 H_4 N_2 O_1$) has a molecular weight of 60. Urea is the source of about half of the antioxidant capacity in the blood. It is produced in the body from the breakdown of proteins.

Restructured Microwater Clusters ($(H_2 O)_5$ to 6) have a typical molecular weight in the range of 90 to 108 for the cluster. Alkaline microwater is enriched in electrons enough to become a reducing agent (antioxidant), delivering free electrons directly into every cell including the optic nerve fibers at the lamina cribrosa to help protect against vision loss associated with glaucoma.

Betaine or Trimethylglycine, usually referred to as TMG ($C5\ H12\ N1$ $O2$) has a molecular weight of 117. TMG is obtained from beets, but for healing purposes, a pure extract allows a therapeutic dose typically up to 3,000 mg a day, and avoids building up excessive iron levels, which would reduce longevity. Pure TMG powder is available from Jarrow.

Taurine ($C2\ H7\ NO3\ S$) has a molecular weight of 125. Taurine is an amino acid that is especially helpful to the retina and heart as an antioxidant. Supplementation is suggested in the form of Magnesium Taurate, available from Cardiovascular Research.

Oxalic Acid ($C2\ H2\ O4$) has a molecular weight of 126 in its hydrated (dihydrate) form. Oxalic acid is found in spinach, taro and rhubarb. We cook these foods to dissolve and remove the oxalic acid. This helps us avoid tissue irritation and deposition of oxalate crystals and stones in the body, and associated problems, which include arthritis. Boil or steam vegetables with oxalic acid content, and discard the water.

Salicylic Acid ($C7\ H6\ O3$) has a molecular weight of 138 (can be obtained in biocompatible complex with bioflavonoids to strengthen blood vessels from willow bark rather than synthetic form in aspirin)

Cinnamic Acid ($C9\ H8\ O2$) has a molecular weight of 148. It is found in cinnamon. Yum. Cinnamon helps stabilize blood sugar regulation. Enjoy it.

N-Acetyl Cysteine, abbreviated NAC ($C_5H_9NO_3S$) has a molecular weight of 163. NAC is a powerful mucolytic, detoxifier and lymphatic drainage remedy. It is a precursor of Glutathione, and supplementation of NAC is the preferred way of raising levels of Glutathione and the crucially important antioxidant enzyme Glutathione Peroxidase (GSH-Px).

Eugenol ($C_{10}H_{12}O_2$) has a molecular weight of 164. Eugenol is found in clove, nutmeg, cinnamon, basil, and bay leaf.

Gallic Acid ($C_7H_6O_5$) has a molecular weight of 170. It is in blackberry, raspberry, walnut, and the medicinal botanicals Boswellia (anti-inflammatory), Triphala (cleansing) and Rhodiola (aerobic metabolism support).

Vitamin C in its ascorbate form ($C_6H_7O_6$) has a molecular weight of 175.

Citric Acid ($C_6H_8O_7$) has a molecular weight of 192. It is in citrus fruits, especially lemons and limes.

Ferulic Acid ($C_{10}H_{10}O_4$) has a molecular weight of 194. Rice bran oil as well as flax and rye are good dietary sources.

Xanthones ($C_{13}H_8O_2$) have a molecular weight of 196. They are in mangosteen, the queen of fruits.

Alpha Lipoic Acid (C8 H14 O2 S2) has a molecular weight of 206. Alpha Lipoic Acid is both fat and water soluble, allowing it to access all intracellular compartments. It is an important recycler of other antioxidants.

Resveratrol (C14 H12 O3) has a molecular weight of 228. It comes from the skins of dark grapes.

Melatonin (C13 H16 N2 O2) has a molecular weight of 232. This hormone is also one of the body's strongest anti-oxidants. It is secreted at night by the pineal gland, which is sensitive to light and electromagnetic fields, so keep electronic devices and wires away from your bed and use a red nightlight or red flashlight if you get up in the middle of the night. Turning on a white light even for a second can stop the pineal from releasing Melatonin for hours or even the rest of the night.

Coral Water Cluster ((H2 O)13 to 15) has a molecular cluster weight of 234-270. Japan has the highest longevity in the world, and Okinawa, where the ground water is naturally filtered through coral, leads the way. Areas with more alkaline water have lower rates of cardiovascular disease (associated with glaucoma) and cancer.

Daidzein (C15 H10 O4) has a molecular weight of 254. Good food sources are kudzu and fermented soy foods like natto, miso and tempeh. Other soy products are better avoided because, like wheat and cow dairy, they contain extremely large protein molecules (gluten in wheat, and casein in cow milk and cow cheese) that are very difficult to digest, and often congest the lymphatic system in the head downstream from the eyes, reducing outflow facility from the eye and thus exacerbating glaucoma.

Pterostilbene (C16 H16 O3) has a molecular weight of 256. It can be enjoyed in blueberries and grapes.

N-Acetyl Carnosine (C11 H16 O4) has a molecular weight of 268 for the Acetyl Carnosine group. It is the most effective way to deliver Carnosine into the eye in eyedrop form, and can also be taken orally for enhanced Carnosine absorption. Carnosine is an important antioxidant dipeptide made of two amino acids, Alanine and Histidine. It is found in brain, muscle and other animal tissues, and because it is only in animals, vegetarians tend to be particularly deficient. Besides scavenging free radicals, Carnosine and N-Acetyl Carnosine also help prevent aging due to formation of Advanced Glycation Endproducts caused by fluctuating sugar levels. It can help in glaucoma by improving microcirculation in the eye.

Genistein (C15 H10 O5) has a molecular weight of 270. It is found in lupins, fava beans, kudzu and fermented soy foods are also suggested sources.

Apigenin (C15 H10 O5) has a molecular weight of 270. It is found in many fruits and vegetables, with celery, parsley and dandelion coffee substitute being excellent sources.

Luteolin (C15 H10 O6) has a molecular weight of 286. Luteolin is in found in green leafy vegetables, as well as celery, green pepper, thyme, chamomile tea, carrots, olive oil, peppermint, rosemary, navel oranges, and oregano.

Cyanidin (C15 H11 O6) has a molecular weight of 287. It is a common red pigment found in grapes, bilberry, blackberry, blueberry, cherry, cranberry, elderberry, hawthorn, acai berry, raspberry, apple, plum, red cabbage and red onion.

Catechin and Epicatechin (C15 H14 O6) both have molecular weights of 290. Recommended sources are acai and peach. Cacao is not recommended due to destabilization of blood sugar, which stresses nerve tissue in glaucoma. Sorry, that means enjoy chocolate treats less often!

Vitamin A: Retinoic Acid form (C20 H28 O2) has a molecular weight of 300.

Ellagic Acid (C14 H6 O8) has a molecular weight of 302. You get it in raspberries and strawberries, but make sure they are organic, especially the strawberries as they retain pesticides particularly well. Pesticides are neurotoxins, developed from wartime nerve gas technologies, so this would be a bad combination with already stressed retinal cells in glaucoma.

Capsaicin (C18 H27 NO3) has a molecular weight of 305. It is the heat in chili peppers.

Gallocatechin, Epigallocatechin (C15 H14 O7) has a molecular weight of 306. Water process decaffeinated extracts of green tea bioflavonoids are suggested rather than higher caffeine containing forms, due to destabilization of blood sugar by caffeine, and the detrimental effect of both hyper and hypoglycemic phases on central nervous system tissue such as the optic nerve fibers in glaucoma. Other sources are banana, persimmon, pomegranate and St. John's wort.

Glutathione (C10 H17 O6 N3 S1) has a molecular weight of 307. Supplementing NAC is the suggested way to increase the body's production of this crucial antioxidant.

Quercetin (C15 H10 O7) has a molecular weight of 338. Onions, citrus, apples and parsley are suggested food sources.

Rosmarinic Acid (C18 H16 O8) has a molecular weight of 360. High levels are available in rosemary, oregano, lemon balm, sage, and marjoram.

Curcumin (C21 H20 O6) has a molecular weight of 368. It is in turmeric.

Vitamin E: Tocopherol form (C29 H50 O2) has a molecular weight of 431. Unique E is the only undiluted, unaltered whole complex vitamin E supplement.

Silymarin (C25 H22 O10) has a molecular weight of 482. It protects the liver in dealing with elimination of toxins. It comes from the botanical medicine milk thistle.

Beta Carotene (C40 H56) has a molecular weight of 536. Fresh carrot juice is an excellent source that has a long history of effective use in healing many chronic degenerative diseases.

Lycopene (C40 H56) has a molecular weight of 537. Fresh vine ripened tomatoes are the best source, with some also found in watermelon and guava.

Theaflavin (C29 H24 O12) has a molecular weight of 564. It is produced by fermentation of green tea into black tea, and also from green tea bioflavonoids as they are processed in the liver. Skip the black tea, and go straight for the bioflavonoids from green tea, minus the caffeine.

Canthaxanthin (C40 H52 O2) has a molecular weight of 565. It is found in mushrooms, algae, crustaceans and fish.

Lutein (C40 H56 O2) has a molecular weight of 569. Lutein is in spinach, kale, Swiss chard, collard greens, beet greens, mustard greens, endive, red pepper and okra)

Zeaxanthin (C40 H56 O2) has a molecular weight of 569. Recommended dietary sources are kale, collard greens, spinach, turnip greens, Swiss chard, mustard greens, beet greens and broccoli.

Naringin (C27 H32 O14) has a molecular weight of 581. Naringin is in grapefruit and one of my favorite fruits: it's larger and sweeter relative, pomelo.

Bilirubin (C33 H36 N4 O6) has a molecular weight of 584. Bilirubin is in the blood from the breakdown of hemoglobin.

Astaxanthin (C40 H52 O4) has a molecular weight of 597. Recommended dietary sources are Pacific or Alaskan salmon. The Atlantic fish are too toxic due to industrial pollution. Supplementation is with BioAstin extracted from red algae grown in Hawaii by Nutrex.

Hesperiden (C28 H34 O15) has a molecular weight of 611. It is found in citrus, and supplementation is suggested as Hesperiden Methyl Chalcone (HMC) for stabilizing mast cells involved in allergic processes related to glaucoma.

Rutin (C27 H30 O16) has a molecular weight of 611. Good dietary sources are buckwheat, asparagus, citrus rinds, mulberries, and cranberries.

Phytic Acid aka Inositol Hexaphosphate or IP6 (C6 H18 O24 P6) has a molecular weight of 660. IP6 is found in seeds and the bran of grains. It chelates minerals making them less bioavailable, so soaking and sprouting are recommended to avoid this effect.

Co-Q10 or Ubiquinone-10 (formula $C_{59} H_{90} O_4$) has a molecular weight of 863. Coenzyme Q10 is synthesized in the body and used in the mitochondria in making cellular energy, especially in tissue with high metabolism; the retina has the highest metabolism of any tissue in the body; the body's production of Co-Q10 is impaired by many beta blockers used to treat glaucoma, as well as blood pressure drugs, and statins for lowering cholesterol, which reduce blood levels as much as 40%; supplementation helps support aerobic cellular metabolism which supplies 95% of the cell's energy needed to maintain visual function and reduce oxidative damage from free radicals)

The various Proanthocyanidin polymers have molecular weights ranging from 1600 to 5500.

Superoxide Dismutase (SOD dimer) is a crucial antioxidant enzyme with a molecular weight of 32,000.

Glutathione Peroxidase (GSH-Px) is another crucial antioxidant enzyme with a higher molecular weight of 95,000.

Catalase (CAT) is a third crucial antioxidant enzyme with an even higher molecular weight of 240,000. The beauty of enzymes is that they can be used over and over again, since they are catalysts that promote quenching of free radicals without getting oxidized in the process, unlike the other antioxidants.

Preventing AGE: Antiglycation

Glycation (sugar deposition) affects both extracellular and intracellular compartments. Glycation can cause amyloid plaque protein deposits, which are classically extracellular, but can also be intracellular. Glycation can also cause aggregation of proteins via cross-linking.

Advanced Glycation Endproducts (AGE) produced by non-enzymatic glycosylation cause cross-linking of collagen and elastin in the connective tissue in the crucial lamina cribrosa, where the delicate optic nerve fibers must pass through a meshwork of connective tissue that is linked to the sclera, the white of the eye that holds the eye's shape. Cross-linking shrinks connective tissue, making us shorter as we age, and increasing the strain on the sensitive optic nerve fibers and their delicate circulation as they pass through the joint-like lamina cribrosa.

AGEs are formed in the body when sugar levels are not stable. They also come in the diet, when we eat cooked carbohydrates. Eating more raw, organic, unprocessed foods is a great start for reducing AGE-ing, along with avoiding things that destabilize sugar regulation, including sugar, alcohol, caffeine, chocolate and stimulants in general. There are also a few nutritional compounds known to protect against AGE formation:

Minerals Vanadium, Chromium and Zinc are involved with sugar regulation and help protect against AGE formation.

Probiotics have been shown to have anti-glycation effects. Probiotics help to produce B vitamins in the gut.

Thiamine (Vitamin B1) reduces AGE generation. High fiber diets tend to supply more thiamine, while thiamine reserves are depleted by alcohol. Garlic and onions supply fat-soluble forms of thiamine (allithiamines) such as benfotiamine, which is more physiologically active than thiamine. Benfotiamine stimulates transketolase, an enzyme essential for normal glucose metabolism, promoting endothelial cell health in the kidney and retina. Benfotiamine helps decrease inflammation and even repair damage that has already taken place to the nerve cells. Benfotiamine supplements are available from Complementary Prescriptions and Source Naturals, with a suggested dosage of 150 mg once or twice a day.

Vitamin B12 helps protect against AGE formation. The recommended form is Methyl Cobalamin, which helps reverse neurological damage.

Vitamin C helps protect against AGE formation. The recommended form is Magnesium Ascorbate. When this form is absorbed by your nerve cells, the Magnesium is drawn in with the Vitamin C. Magnesium is beneficial inside the cell, while Calcium is not.

Vitamin E helps protect against AGE formation. The recommended form is Unique E, the only pure, unadulterated Vitamin E complex supplement on the market since 1963 available only through nutritional physicians (made by AC Grace). Unique E is much more therapeutic than other forms of Vitamin E. It can be safely taken at higher dosages, although it is always recommended to taper up Vitamin E dosages gradually so that blood pressure is not destabilized. Unique, unlike other fat-soluble vitamin E products, is stable against oxidation at room temperature. This means it will be more stable at body temperature, too! Other companies dilute their Vitamin E in soy oil.

The active co-enzyme form of Vitamin B6, Pyridoxal 5' Phosphate (P5P) reduces AGE formation, and is widely available as a supplement from many manufacturers. Pyridoxamine, a relative of Vitamin B6, also reduces AGE formation, especially fat derived AGEs, though not as well as P5P. Pyridoxamine reduces AGE levels, preventing complications of aging and diabetes as documented in animal studies. It is found in carrots, walnuts, fish and chicken, and used to be available over the counter as a vitamin supplement, but the FDA has forced it off the market so it can potentially be regulated as a more expensive drug in the future.

The currently available prescription anti-diabetic medication Metformin (Glucophage) does reduce AGE formation. The investigative new drugs Pimagedine (aminoguanidine) and Alagebrium were also being tested for anti-glycation effects but are not on the market.

Bioflavonoids are also called Vitamin P. Resveratrol from the skin of red grapes as well as cranberries and blueberries, has protective anti-glycation effects. Other bioflavonoids in cinnamon, clove, yerba mate and green tea reportedly have anti-glycation effects. Cinnamon and clove both improve blood sugar regulation, so enjoy! Yerba mate and green tea have beneficial bioflavonoids that could be useful as exracts, but avoidance of the stimulant effects of the drinking tea made from the whole herb is recommended. Caffeine free extracts of Camelia sinensis (green tea) containing the beneficial bioflavonoids called catechins and epigallocatechin gallates (EGCG) are available and are recommended. Oral EGCG attenuates injury to the retina caused by ischemia/reperfusion. Light induced apoptosis is also reduced. (Zhang B, Rusciano D, Osborne NN. Orally administered epigallocatechin gallate attenuates retinal neuronal death in vivo and light-induced apoptosis in vitro.)

N-Acetyl Carnosine (an antioxidant found in animal tissues, and thus deficient in vegetarians) acts as a scavenger to inhibit AGE formation, preventing protein modification, protecting LDL from both AGE and oxidation, and even reversing damage that has already occurred. N-Acetyl Carnosine is available as an oral nutritional supplement and is additionally supplied directly in eye-drop form. Carnosine is less bio-available, but also available as a supplement, and dosages of 1,000 to

1,500 mg per day are recommended. Beta-Alanine, one of the amino acid components of the dipeptide Carnosine, is another option to help reverse AGE, since dosages of 1,000 mg twice a day help the retinal cells produce increased levels of Carnosine.

Alpha-Lipoic Acid, found in potato, carrot, broccoli, beet and yam also helps prevent AGE formation. Alpha-Lipoic Acid is an excellent nutritional supplement with many additional benefits as it regenerates other antioxidants including Vitamin C.

Minerals

Calcium

Calcium, when mishandled, can constrict blood vessels. Calcium supplementation often helps to improve calcium handling. Excess calcium, however is linked to arterial-vascular disease.

Chromium & Vanadium

Depleted chromium levels in body tissues are related to increases in IOP with visual stress. A combination of low dietary chromium, due to the loss of this trace mineral in food refining, together with the loss of this mineral when eating sugar and refined foods, or foods high in vanadium, results in increasing the risk of elevated IOP by 4.7 times. It is well documented that chromium stores in Americans are generally depleted with aging, due to our diet high in sugar and refined carbohydrates. It is also well known that glaucoma incidence also increases dramatically with age. Since age itself is not a potential cause, being merely the passage of time, in the course of which causality may occur, we should be looking for more factors like chromium, heavy metals, and free radical effects at the optic nerve head to understand and prevent glaucoma. Vanadium should be avoided as it antagonizes chromium. Vanadium is more concentrated in low fat dairy products, seaweed, mushrooms, vinegar, chocolate, carob, poultry and large fish (tuna, swordfish and shark), while more chromium is found in red meats, whole grains, molasses, fruits, vegetables, eggs (in the yolk) and dairy products made from whole milk.

Chromium improves lipid profiles. Recommended forms of chromium for supplementation are either chromium picolinate or chromium polynicotinate, and not 'amino acid chelated' chromium, which can contain large unlabeled amounts of vanadium. A dosage of 200 to 600 mcg/day is recommended especially if taking topical or oral beta-blockers to counteract their detrimental effects of lipid metabolism. 600 mcg/day increased HDL levels 16% to 38% in people on oral beta-blockers, resulting in 12 to 17% reduction in the risk of heart disease.

Copper

Excess or unnecessary copper should be avoided, as in excess it promotes free radical pathology.

Germanium

Germanium (100 to 200 mg/day) can help relieve discomfort associated with certain types of glaucoma, as it increases delivery of needed oxygen to the nerve cells.

Iron

Excess or unnecessary iron should be avoided, as in excess it promotes free radical pathology.

Magnesium

Magnesium may be beneficial in preventing mishandling of calcium, which can lead to vasospasms in the optic nerve. This could be especially important in low-tension glaucoma, where it is being suggested that calcium channel blockers might be used to produce this effect. Calcium channel blockers have been shown to increase peripheral vision in people with cold hands. Calcium channel blockers have been found to prevent the progression of optic nerve damage in 100% of glaucoma patients. The problem with calcium channel blocker drugs is their side effects. Magnesium is nature's calcium channel blocker, increasing cyclic AMP levels through inhibition of calcium influx into the cell, resulting in relaxation of smooth muscle as well as prevention of platelet aggregation. Smooth muscles control the drainage of fluid from the eye. Cyclic AMP is also the primary intracellular regulator of aqueous humor production and IOP. Magnesium is 85% depleted in farmland soils, as this macromineral is not present in the commercial NPK (nitrogen, phosphorus and potassium) fertilizer preparations. As a result, 80% of adults are deficient in Magnesium. Magnesium deficiency is linked to high blood pressure, which in turn is associated with glaucoma. Even patients on oral beta-blockers can reduce blood pressure by taking 365 mg/day of Magnesium. 750 mg/day of Magnesium has been shown to improve retinal circulation in patients with hypertensive retinopathy and 243 mg/day improved both circulation and visual fields in glaucoma patients with vasospasm. Magnesium can reverse atrial fibrillation, which is linked to low-tension glaucoma. Low Magnesium intake is also linked to deaths from sudden heart attack, making repletion to optimal levels critical in the American population. Low Magnesium combined with high Calcium promotes coagulation of the blood as well as increases in adrenal hormones that increase IOP. Magnesium glycinate is the most absorbable form of magnesium, and generally does not result in diarrhea as other less well-absorbed forms do in therapeutic dosages. It may take up to about 6 months to rebuild a deficient magnesium level, so it is important not to give up if there is no apparent immediate benefit. People with Raynaud's disease (cold extremeties), a condition linked to low-tension glaucoma, for example do not respond as rapidly as healthy adults to Magnesium supplements. Stress, a condition, which has been linked to glaucoma, increases the demand for Magnesium. The average American does not even consume the RDA level of Magnesium. A dosage of 250 to 400 mg/day at bedtime has been recommended at a 1:1 ratio with Calcium. It is often suggested to take Calcium at a different time of day to maximize absorption of both Calcium and Magnesium, since they are both divalent cations and thus compete for the same absorption channels. Magnesium glycinate is the most absorbable form of

Magnesium, eliminating the common side effect of diarrhea often experienced with high doses of Magnesium. As Magnesium levels are repleted over a period of about 6 months, watch for improvements in visual fields, visual acuity and circulation to the optic nerve. Watch also for muscular weakness as a possible indication that Magnesium levels have been built up higher than necessary. Higher Magnesium levels may be needed when taking higher levels of Calcium, and when taking diuretic medications.

Manganese

Manganese supplementation at 20 mg/day has been suggested as part of a total nutritional program for glaucoma. Manganese picolinate is a bioavailable form.

Zinc

Zinc supplementation with zinc picolinate or zinc monomethionine is often recommended, and a simple taste test using Zinc Sulfate solution can be used to monitor the degree of deficiency as well as the response to supplementation. A dosage of 15 to 25 mg/day of zinc has been recommended.

Vitamins & Cofactors

Nutrition in Glaucoma

A good step in developing a balanced foundation for your nutritional program is to begin with a broad-spectrum multi-nutrient supplement. A multiple to be used by someone with glaucoma should have both vitamin A and beta-carotene according to some doctors. Rapid and sustained pressure reductions of 5 to 7 mm Hg have been achieved in studies using improved diet with supplementation of nutrients including vitamins A, B1, B2, B3, B5, and calcium, which is better than results achieved with current medical therapy. Malnutrition and malabsorption syndromes should also be ruled out or treated, as they may contribute to optic nerve damage and susceptibility. Glaucoma in a malnourished population was brought under control within one week with the antioxidants 180,000 I.U./day of vitamin A, 200 I.U./day of vitamin E and 3,000 mg/day of vitamin C.

Vitamin A and carotenoids

Vitamin A deficiency has been observed in the glaucoma population. Blood levels of carotenoids (pro-vitamin A) are lower in people with glaucoma than in normals. Vitamin A is necessary to prevent hydration and swelling of the collagen in the drainage angle of the eye, which can block outflow. Loss of xanthophyll carotenoids in the papillo-macular area is the first detectable indication of loss of optic nerve fibers in glaucoma. Some practitioners recommend 25,000 IU/day of natural source beta-carotene or a combination of vitamin A and beta-carotene (pro-vitamin A) along with 400 IU/day of either dry or mixed tocopherol vitamin E. Beta-carotene dosages up to 30 mg/day have been suggested as safe by the Alliance for Aging Research. Others recommend up to 40,000 IU/day of beta-carotene.

Vitamin B Complex

The entire B complex, with specific emphasis on vitamins B1, B3, B5 B6, B12, folate, inositol and choline (or lecithin, as a source of choline) may be particularly helpful in glaucoma. A 50 mg B complex taken 3 times a day with meals is a good base, and in some cases B vitamin injections (preferably unpreserved) may be needed.

B1

Thiamine (Vitamin B1) deficiency causes optic nerve disease and is depleted by stress. Optic atrophy linked to thiamine deficiency can be reversed in 10 days with large supplemental doses. Thiamine may be poorly absorbed and metabolized, or otherwise demanded at increased levels in glaucoma patients, as they usually have reduced blood levels despite normal dietary intake. This has been associated with lack of digestive enzymes resulting in malabsorption. A dosage of 25 to 50 mg a day has been recommended, except for smokers who should take 300 mg/day until vision improves.

B3

Vitamin B3 cleans out the capillaries, reversing the effects of arteriosclerosis that contributes to glaucoma. B3 also dilates the capillaries, further improving blood flow to and from the eye and optic nerve. B3 raises ATP levels in depleted cells, raising their resistance to stressors like glutamate, which is associated with glaucoma.

B5

Vitamin B5 (100 mg taken 3 times a day) helps to strengthen the adrenal glands.

B6

Vitamin B6 decreases IOP by its diuretic effect. A dosage of 25 to 50 mg/day is recommended.

B12

B12 may be preventive in low-tension glaucoma. Vitamin B12 deficiency, pernicious anemia, can by itself cause damage to the optic nerve. Over one million American seniors have pernicious anemia.

The first sign of deficiency in over half of Vitamin B12 deprived animals is damage to the myelin sheath of the papillomacular bundle. In humans, too, B12 deficiency is linked to demyelinating processes like multiple sclerosis. Fortunately, resulting vision loss has been shown to be mostly reversible with B12 supplementation. B12 actually supports regeneration of the myelin sheath. In humans, neurological damage including vision loss and optic atrophy are often seen before anemia is detected. Visual disorders associated with alcohol and tobacco clear up with Vitamin B12. Borderline B12 status may contribute to the susceptibility of the optic nerve to damage from other metabolic stress factors, and optic nerve damage from early B12 deficiency can precede any measurable changes in the blood. Pallor of the optic nerve head, considered a sign of glaucoma, is also a classic result of pernicious anemia. This is frequently accompanied by hypochlorhydria, leading to poor assimilation of many minerals and other glaucoma-preventive nutrients, and IOP may be either normal or increased. Over half of seniors lack adequate hydrochloric acid secretion to absorb B12 efficiently. B12 deficiency can cause nervous system related symptoms including memory loss, confusion, dementia, depression and psychosis, all seen more frequently in the elderly. B12 deficiency is also accompanied frequently by photophobia and dependency on sun-wear, as is deficiency of other B vitamins, as well as vitamin A and zinc. One 5-year study showed that 1500 mcg/day of vitamin B12 stopped the progression of visual field loss in glaucoma, and a significant percentage of patients actually had some vision restored. Since there was no change in eye pressure with B12 supplementation, different levels of B12, which can be stored in the body for years, may explain why some people can sustain higher pressures without damage to the optic nerve. Numerous studies confirm the beneficial effects of B12 supplementation on optic nerve disease. Supplementation may be especially beneficial when initiated within 6 months of the onset of visual symptoms. Coffee and aspirin are factors, which impair vitamin B12 absorption. Zinc, which is necessary for production of hydrochloric acid, and digestive enzymes are recommended for some individuals to aid B12 absorption. A suggested dosage of 1500 to 2500 mcg/day of vitamin B12 has been proposed, as contrasted with the average adult intake of 5 mcg/day. Intramuscular injections may also be necessary initially for smokers and those with hypochlorhydria. Unpreserved injections are far preferable if they can be obtained. The hydroxycobalamin form has been shown to be effective when cyanocobalamin was not. The preferred form for reversing neurological conditions is Methylcobalamin. The caution with Methylcobalamin is that it is the catalyst for methylation of Mercury, so Dibencozide, the active coenzyme form of vitamin B12 in the mitochondria, is an important alternative or complement to consider.

Folate

Folate may be preventive in low-tension glaucoma. Folate is high in raw, fresh salad vegetables such as asparagus, spinach leaves, garbanzo beans, and bean sprouts, as well as fresh, ripe, raw fruits. This means that it is important to find sources for locally grown organic produce, since folate is the least stable and most often deficient of all vitamins in this country. 400 mcg per day has been recommended, with 1000 mcg a day suggested for smokers.

Choline

Choline (1,000 to 2,000 mg/day) cleans out the capillaries along with Vitamin B3, reversing the effects of arteriosclerosis that contributes to glaucoma. Others have recommended at least 100 mg/day.

Inositol

Inositol is important in reducing stress that can trigger increased IOP.

TMG

Trimethylglycine (TMG) is the most efficient methyl donor, providing three methyl groups per molecule. This is crucial in reversing atherosclerosis, and thus restoring adequate circulation to the retina. TMG recycles homocysteine, associated with elevated cardiovascular risk much more strongly than is cholesterol, to SAMe.

Vitamin C

People who consume vitamin C ($\leq$ 100 mg/day) have significantly lower odds of glaucoma compared with those who consumed no vitamin C (odds ratio: OR = 0.34; 95% confidence interval: CI = 0.13-0.87). This correlation was also significant at the highest quartile dosage of vitamin C (>900 mg/day; adjusted OR = 0.47; 95% CI = 0.23-0.97).

Vitamin C reduces intraocular pressure (IOP), according to research at the University of Rome. Daily intake of 35 grams in divided doses was used for patients weighing 150 pounds, with adjustments in this dosage proportional to body weight. Rapid and significant drops in pressure were obtained. A single dose of 500 mg/kg (about 35 grams for a 150 pound person) resulted significantly lowered IOP in 100% of patients, by an average of 16 mm Hg. Unfortunately, at such a high dosage, using the acid form of vitamin C causes diarrhea in may people, so neutral pH ascorbate or polyascorbate (ester) vitamin C is recommended by the author. Doses of up to 2 to 10 grams may be taken 4 times a day. Over 90% of patients given 100 to 150 mg/kg ascorbic acid 3 to 5 times a day achieved essentially normal IOP within 45 days, with GI symptoms only persisting for 3 to 4 days. Some of these patients had previously uncontrollable IOP even when taking maximum medical therapy. On the other end of the dosage spectrum, even low levels of vitamin C, such as 1200 mg/day have been shown to reduce IOP, when compared to a near RDA level of 75 mg/day, with a high level of statistical significance ($p < .001$). A study using .5 gm of ascorbic acid 4 times a day showed significant decreases in IOP after 6 days. Another study showed that .5 gm twice a day for 1 week significantly reduced IOP, which returned to the previous baseline level after 1 week off the vitamin C supplement. Even eye drops made of 10% ascorbic acid used 3 times a day for 3 days significantly lowered IOP of the treated eye compared to patients' other untreated eye. Vitamin C is accepted as a treatment for glaucoma in European and Asian countries. One advantage of vitamin C over drugs therapies is that vitamin C not only lowers IOP through a combination of increased blood osmolarity, decreased aqueous production and improved outflow, but it also provides anti-oxidant protection and enhances impaired collagen metabolism, which appears to be the primary cause of glaucoma. Vitamin C helps to regenerate type I collage, laminin and fibronectin in the trabecular meshwork. A month of topical steroid treatment lowers vitamin C levels by over 50% in the aqueous humor, over 60% in the vitreous humor and nearly 85% in the lens. Thousands of people get cataracts and/or glaucoma while on steroid therapies each year, yet few doctors recommend increased intakes of vitamin C for prevention. One author recommends at least 500 to 1000 mg/day of Vitamin C, and 2000 to 3000 mg/day for smokers.

See also: Feldman RM, Steinmann WC, Spaeth GL et al: Oral ascorbic acid in the treatment of glaucoma. Glaucoma 1987; 19(6): 181-183.

Bioflavonoids

Rutin

Rutin, a bioflavonoid, supplemented at 60 mg/day in divided doses reduced IOP by at least 15% in 17 out of 26 eyes with uncomplicated primary glaucoma. These patients were also found to respond better to drug treatment following at least one month on rutin supplementation, as well. Some practitioners now recommend a dosage of 50 mg 3 times a day of Rutin. Mixed bioflavonoids should be taken at a dosage of 1,000 mg/day for all types of glaucoma. Bioflavonoids (which are also active components of herbs such as ginkgo and bilberry, in the herb section) have been shown to further reduce IOP in patients on miotic drops.

Quercetin

Quercetin inhibits histamine release. It also increases cyclic AMP, relaxing smooth muscle. In addition, it is an effective oral chelation agent for removing excess iron that contributes to free radical pathology. Quercetin has been recommended at a dosage from 500 mg/day up to 3000 mg/day.

Quercetin Dihydrate

Water-soluble Quercetin Dihydrate maximizes absorption, making it more clinically effective and more cost effective than the common form. Potentially therapeutic dosages can be found in Pain Guard Forte' (from Perque) with 500 mg per tablet, and Aller-C (from Vital Nutrients) with 250 mg per capsule, along with synergistic Vitamin C and citrus bioflavonoids. Therapeutic dosages range up to 4 grams (8 tablets or 16 capsules) a day in chronic conditions, while up to 8 grams (16 tablets or 32 capsules) a day may be needed for relief of acute pain and inflammatory processes such as in acute glaucoma attacks. Bowel tolerance (resulting in loose stool) may be reached in the capsule form at acute therapeutic dosages due to the ascorbic acid content.

Apigenin

Apigenin (4',5,7-trihydroxyflavone from celery, parsley, dandelion coffee, chamomile and other vegetables and fruits) has healing properties that include antiangioneogenesis and nerve regeneration, as well as stress-reducing anxiolytic and slight sedative effects. Adult neurogenesis has been demonstrated both in vitro and in vivo in an animal model. (Taupin, P. Apigenin and related compounds stimulate adult neurogenesis. Mars, Inc., the Salk Institute for Biological Studies: WO2008147483.) Typical therapeutic dosages range from 25 to 50 mg per day and therapeutic dosages are available in a B Complex Stress

Formula from Pioneer, as well as Life Extension's Triple Action Cruciferous Vegetable Extract.

Vitamin D

Vitamin D may also be beneficial. The best source of this vitamin is moderate daily exposure to sunlight and the use of full spectrum lighting indoors. It is important to note that excess dietary calcium, vitamin A and vitamin D3(25,OH) from diets high in vitamin A & D fortified commercial dairy products may actually be a contributor to low-tension glaucoma.

Vitamin E

Vitamin E has been recommended in combination with ginkgo biloba or with vitamins A and C. Dosages of 400 IU/day have been recommended, with smokers requiring double that level. Others also suggest safe dosages of vitamin E up to 800 I.U./day. Esterified natural dry vitamin E (succinate), which I call 'Ester E' has been shown to be easier on the liver to absorb and process in research by Jeffrey Bland, Ph.D., President of Health-Comm. The only oil form of vitamin E that is undiluted by vegetable oil and therefore stable against oxidation is Unique E.

Nutritional-Cofactors

Coenzyme Q10

CoQ10 can improve impaired heart function, improving the quality of circulation, which is especially important in low pressure glaucoma. Together with Vitamin E, CoQ10 has proven beneficial in glaucoma. CoQ10 raises ATP levels in depleted cells, reducing risk of damage by glutamate. A daily dose of at least 30 mg/day of CoQ10, increased to 100 mg/day for low-tension glaucoma, has been recommended.

PQQ

Another important quinone is Pyrroloquinoline Quinone. PQQ is the only supplement known to stimulate mitochondrial regeneration. The only other method that can achieve this revitalization of oxidative cellular metabolism involves prolonged and severe calorie intake restriction.

Alpha Lipoic Acid

150 mg daily of alpha lipoic acid has been reported to improve visual function in patients with open angle glaucoma in stages I and II.

Essential Fatty Acids

Essential fatty acids, precursors of anti-inflammatory prostaglandins, may be very beneficial in reducing chronic inflammatory processes involved in glaucoma. Eskimos who have a high intake of omega-3 fatty acids from fish have a very low incidence of open angle glaucoma. Fish oil supplements have also been found beneficial in Raynaud's syndrome, which is related to low-tension glaucoma. The typical American diet is deficient in omega-3 fatty acids. Depleted levels of the omega-3 fatty acid eicosapentaenoic acid, or EPA, can be supplemented with dietary small cold-water fish (salmon, mackerel, sardines, herring, cod) and fish oil capsules. This common deficiency is a suspected risk factor for both pigmentary and low-tension forms of glaucoma. Omega-3 oils thin the blood, improving circulation. They have also been shown to produce significant lowering of IOP in rabbits. Even diabetics can take up to 2.5 grams of EPA without any side effects. Other sources of the beneficial omega 3 fatty acids include black currant oil, as well as flax or hemp seeds or their oils. Omega-6 oils are also important. Diabetics have impaired omega-6 metabolism, contributing to demyelination of nerves. Beneficial omega-6 oils are available as evening primrose oil and borage oil. Deficiency of both omega-3 and omega-6 oils are linked to pigmentary glaucoma. In opposition to the beneficial fatty acids are long-chain and trans-fatty acids found in fried foods and hydrogenated oils such as margarine. These junk and processed foods should be avoided as they promote inflammatory processes and probably increase the risk of pigmentary glaucoma as well as many other diseases systemically. A suggested dosage of omega-3 fish oil, flax or hemp seed oil is at least 1000 mg/day. Omega-6 fatty acids double cyclic AMP levels, and when combined with *Coleus forskohlii* or its extract, Forskolin, triple these levels (see herb section). A combined dosage of omega-3 and omega-6 oils is recommended at 500 to 3000 mg/day.

Immune Modulators: Phytosterols & Others

Phytosterols

Phytosterols, such as beta sitosterol, are plant fats, related in structure to cholesterol, but functioning as immune modulators. This means that they reduce problematic inflammatory responses to toxins and allergens, while increasing immunity against pathogens. They are found at high levels in sprouts, and have traditionally been filtered out of virtually all commercial oils to make them clear and visually attractive for increased sales. Unfiltered flax oil is now available in health food stores.

Therapeutic levels of plant sterols are available in Sterol Max (from Enriching Gifts) and ModuCare (licensed by Wakunaga through a variety of manufacturers including Thorne Research).

Probiotics

Probiotic gut flora and symbionts are crucial immune modulators. There should be approximately 2 pounds of the friendly flora in the gut. This is not the case in modern populations because the beneficial flora are destroyed by coffee, toxins, antibiotics, the flu, and many other stressors.

Magnesium

Magnesium is an essential immune modulator needed as a coenzyme for 300 different processes throughout the body. Deficiency is linked to immune dysfunction, and is found in 70 to 95 percent of the modern population, because it has been mined out of the soils by modern agribusiness methods. Vegetables have lost 25-80% since the middle of the 20th century, and refining of grains removes 80-95%. Magnesium was traditionally re-supplied to field crops by spreading manure, but modern chemical fertilizers are limited to NPK (Nitrogen, Phosphorus & Potassium) because crops still grow as large without the other macro and trace minerals that are essential to our health. Magnesium Glycinate is the best-absorbed form for repletion, and Magnesium Taurate is often recommended in glaucoma since taurine acts as an antioxidant in the retina and the heart.

IP6

Inositol hexaphosphate (IP6), also known as phytate, is an immunomodulator, but can deplete important nutrient minerals when taken long term, so be sure to follow with mineral supplementation. IP6 is found in beans, brown rice, corn, sesame seeds, wheat bran, and many fiber-rich foods.

Vitamin D3

Besides being an important neurohormone, Vitamin D3 is an essential immune modulator made from Cholesterol when exposed to natural sunlight without interference by sunscreens. Many drugs deplete D3 and deficiency is linked to autoimmune disorders. If your level is low and your liver is making extra Cholesterol, this may be your body's best attempt to restore levels. Take a high potency D3 supplement to restore above average levels.

Botanicals

Herbs well documented as immunomodulators both in vitro and in vivo include:

Shatavari (*Asparagus racemosus*)

Neem (*Azadirachta indica*)

Holy basil (*Ocimum sanctum*)

Ginseng (*Panax ginseng*)

Picrorhiza (*Picrorhiza kurroa*)

Guduchi (*Tinospora cordifolia*)

Ashwagandha (*Withania somnifera*)

(Agarwal, SS and Singh, VK. Immunomodulators: A Review of Studies on Indian Medicinal Plants and Synthetic Peptides, Part I: Medicinal Plants)

Curcumin

Curcumin is the major component in turmeric (*Curcuma longa*), a member of the ginger family. It is anti-inflammatory and inhibits autoimmune reactions, and its capacity as an immunomodulator has been documented both in vitro and in vivo. Piperine in black pepper and coconut milk both help increase absorption from foods, and some supplements are specially designed to increase bio-availability.

Olive leaf extract

Olive (*Olea europea*) leaf extract contains Oleuropein, a patented immunomodulator.

Blackseed oil

Blackseed oil (Nigella sativa) is an immunomodulator. Muhammad said that blackseed is a "cure for everything but death".

Oleander extract

Oleander is an immune stimulator and modulator. The raw plant is toxic, so stick to prepared extracts.

Mushrooms

Many mushrooms have important immunomodulating effects with the most important being A. brasiliensis (Royal sun agaricus, or Himematsutake), which contains Flo-a-beta and FA-2-b-Md, C. volvatus, which contains H-3-B, and F. velutipes (Winter mushroom, or Enokitake) containing Flammulin. (Evid Based Complement Alternat Med. 2005 September; 2(3): 285–299. PMCID: PMC1193547)

Colostrum and Transfer Factor

Immune factors are intensively transferred to offspring by mammals in the first day or two of milk production. This first milk is known as colostrum, and it contains Transfer Factor. Bovine source works for humans, but should be from healthy organically raised cows, and preferably collected in the first 24 hours.

MGN3

MGN3 Biobran is a potent and well-documented mushroom-based immunomodulator.

Amino Acids & Polypeptides

Amino Acids

Acetyl-L-Carnitine (ALC) raises ATP energy levels in neurons. It is neuroprotective against the excitatory amino acid glutamate, which is elevated in glaucoma. L-Arginine relaxes the smooth muscle in blood vessels. It also supports regeneration of the myelin sheath along with adenosyl methionine and polyamines. Glutathione is a tripeptide, which helps prevent oxidative damage to the trabecular meshwork. In animal research, trabecular outflow was only reduced with suppression of the glutathione antioxidant system. Oxidation of the methionine present in collagen in the trabecular meshwork of glaucomatous human eyes has been observed. N-acetyl cysteine, a glutathione precursor, is recommended at supplemental doses of 200 to 600 mg/day. Methyl-sulfonyl methane, a source of organic sulfur, may help to raise glutathione levels. Reduced glutathione is also available as a supplement. Glutathione increases ATP energy levels in nerve cells, protecting against damage by Glutamate. L-Carnosine provides neuroprotection via antioxidant activity and independent defense against excitotoxins. L-Carnosine raises Glutathione levels.

N-Acetyl L-Tyrosine

L-Tyrosine is important for the formation of epinephrine, norepinephrine, dopamine and serotonin. N-Acetyl L-Tyrosine is a rapidly absorbed, highly bio-available form of L-Tyrosine, providing greater therapeutic benefits at lower dosages. Tyrosine is not an essential amino acid, because the body can make limited quantities from the essential amino acid L-Phenylalanine. L-Tyrosine is the starting point for the body to sequentially make the catecholamine neurotransmitters L-DOPA, dopamine, norepinephrine, and finally epinephrine (which is commonly used to treat glaucoma; see neurotransmitter section). When epinephrine is made it uses up a methyl group from SAMe, leaving it as homocysteine which is a major contributor to cardiovascular disease. SAMe can be regenerated by other methyl donors in the B vitamin family, such as folate, B6 and B12, but the methyl donors are our culture's leading vitamin deficiency, due to lack of fresh greens from kitchen gardens. The most efficient solution for this is Trimethyl Glycine (TMG), a triple methyl donor in the B vitamin and amino acid families, extracted from beets (avoiding excessive iron, which shortens lifespan).

A cost effective combination of Forskolin and N-acetyl L-Tyrosine is available from Cardiovascular Research. TMG is available as a pure water-soluble powder from Jarrow. The amino acid Glycine is named for its slightly sweet taste, so TMG can even be taken straight in the mouth if you find it fairly pleasant tasting, as I do.

Communication Molecules:
Hormones, Prostaglandins &
Neurotransmitters

Adrenal Gland & Corticosteroids

Epinephrine is a natural neuro-hormone, released by the adrenal glands, which is often used to treat glaucoma in conventional medicine. Adrenal glandulars, including adrenal cortex and other nutritional supports for rebuilding the adrenal function should be used whenever the adrenals are run down. Vitamin C and the B complex are particularly important for supporting the adrenals. Adrenal hormones seem to be the primary daytime regulators of IOP. Among the natural over the counter (OTC) hormones used to restore adrenal function are Pregnenolone, Progesterone, DHEA and 7-Keto DHEA. 7-Keto has the advantage of not affecting sex hormone production. Estrogen can also affect IOP regulation.

Cortisol is a stress related adrenal hormone. High cortisol contributes to glaucoma and can cause elevation of blood sugar, blood pressure, and intraocular pressure (IOP). The preferred remedy for elevated cortisol is frequent laughter. Botanical adaptagens and compounds to support reduction in stress responses and cortisol levels include

Cortisol Manager (Integrative Therapeutics), Relora (a proprietary combination of *Magnolia officinalis* and *Phelodendron amurense* available in various labels), Ashwagandha (*Withania somnifera*), *Eleutherococcus senticosus* (Siberian ginseng), schisandra (Magnolia vine) and *Rhodiola rosea*.

Pineal Gland & Melatonin

Melatonin, the hormone of darkness, secreted by the pineal gland, seems to be the primary nighttime regulator of IOP. Many glaucoma patients also manifest sleep disturbances. Melatonin is significantly associated with longevity, cancer prevention and restful sleep, as well. Its production can be blocked by turning a light turned on or left on during sleep or when waking during the night, as well as by electromagnetic and geopathic field exposure. Using a red filter over a flashlight or nightlight preserves the pineals ability to sustain melatonin production. Melatonin may be taken as a supplement before bedtime, or alternatively, its production seems to be enhanced by stimulating the retina with violet light for up to 20 minutes before sleep. Melatonin reduces the rate of aqueous production from the daytime level of 3.1 microliters/minute to 1.5 microliters/minute during sleep. IOP, with a daily rhythm of changing pressure normally fluctuating about 5 to 7 mm of Hg (and more in many glaucoma patients), typically peaks just after waking. This is also when brain temperature and cerebral circulation peak, stimulated by light entering the eyes. Taken during the daytime, however, Melatonin has detrimental effects, promoting

112

cancer in animal studies, and shows no effect on the rate of aqueous fluid production.

Thyroid Gland & Thyroxin

Thyroid glandulars or thyroid hormone replacement therapy can be helpful. Thyroid activity, along with zinc, is needed to metabolize beta-carotene into vitamin A for the eyes. Both thyroid and adrenal regulation is needed to support the high-energy metabolism of the cells in the retina, which have a higher metabolic rate than any other tissue in the body. When thyroxine is prescribed medically, the natural source (Armour thyroid) is preferable to synthetic (Synthroid), as electrodermal measures show better tolerance by the liver, which according to principles of oriental medicine is known to exert a strong influence on eye conditions.

Prostaglandins

Melatonin is the only molecular communicator that directly enters every cell in the body, synchronizing the diurnal and seasonal rhythms of all systems to work together coherently. Prostaglandins carry the messages of all other hormones within the cells, and also play an important role in regulating IOP, circulation and inflammation responses.

Regulating intra-cellular communication via prostaglandins has demonstrated superior diurnal IOP control over all other glaucoma medications. The botanical medicine *Coleus forskohlii* also regulates intra-cellular communication via c-AMP, which mediates most of the effects of prostaglandin PGE 2.

Endogenous physiologic signaling receptors, prostaglandins, actions and pathways:

DP1-2 receptors bind to PGD 2 and increase Ca^{++} via PLC stimulation.

EP1 receptors bind to prostaglandin PGE 2 and increase Ca^{++} via PLC stimulation.

EP2 receptors bind to prostaglandin PGE 2 and increase cAMP via AC stimulation.

EP3 receptors bind to prostaglandin PGE 2 and decrease cAMP via AC inhibition.

EP4 receptors bind to prostaglandin PGE 2 and increase cAMP via AC stimulation.

FP receptors bind to prostaglandin PGF 2 and increase Ca^{++} via PLC stimulation.

IP1-2 receptors bind to prostaglandin PGI 2 and increase Ca^{++} via PLC stimulation.

TP receptors bind to prostaglandin TxA 2 and increase Ca^{++} via PLC stimulation.

Don't worry... you won't be tested on this. You don't have to memorize it! As Einstein said, when asked by a reporter why he couldn't remember Maxwell's equations, "I know where to look it up!"

The point here is that your cells have intricate mechanisms of intracellular communication based on essential fatty acids that regulate functions like inflammation and smooth muscle relaxation which in turn regulates local circulation. So let's take a closer look at a few of these pathways that are important in glaucoma.

Eicosanoids, precursors, related analogs, and local physiologic actions

Prostaglandin PGD 3 is made from Omega-3 essential fatty acids EPA & DHA, which can be made by the body in limited amounts from plant precursors. PGD 3 lowers IOP without inflammatory effects (rabbit). This is a very beneficial pathway to support with high quality fish oil supplements that are assayed to assure they are free of toxins including heavy metals that accumulate in larger fish, especially today's in polluted waters.

Prostaglandin PGE 2 is made from Arachidonic acid, which is high in the modern diet, and is chemically related to the synthetic analogs (imitations) latanoprost (Xalatan), travoprost (Travatan), bimatoprost (Lumigan) and unoprostone isopropyl (Rescula). PGE 2 stimulates hyperalgesic response (sensitizes to pain), promotes inflammation (which activates local tissue cleansing, but can also contribute to tissue damage) and lowers IOP. This communication pathway, which tends to be over-stimulated in our culture, is like a double-edged sword with the potential to lower IOP, which does not guarantee protection against damage, and the potential to increase inflammatory tissue damage.

Prostaglandin PGE 3 is made from Omega-3 essential fatty acids EPA and DHA and indirectly in limited quantities from plant precursors. PGE 3 lowers IOP without inflammatory effects (rabbit). Like PGD 3, this pathway is supported by high quality fish oil supplements of documented purity.

The prostaglandin PGF 2 is made from PGE 2. PGF 2 lowers IOP and inhibits inflammation by raising levels of cyclic Adenosine Monophosphate (cAMP).

Forskolin, in the botanical medicine *Coleus forskohlii,* works on the PGE 2 pathway by raising cAMP levels as well, reducing risk of associated tissue damage from processes like free radical pathology, collagen cross-linking and reduction of circulatory perfusion of optic nerve tissues. In fact, where many prescription eye drops risk side effects in those with heart and lung issues, Forskolin, like the Omega 3 EFAs, has side benefits, and can even be used to treat these problems.

Most anti-inflammatory drug therapies try to block pro-inflammatory physiological pathways. Prednisone, which can cause glaucoma even in eye drop or skin cream forms, is used in high doses to block the liberation of arachidonic acid, the precursor of the pro-inflammatory prostaglandins. This can usually be more safely achieved with supplementation of the safer (OTC) steroids DHEA, its active metabolite 7-Keto, or its precursor pregnenolone, as well as immune-modulating plant-analog phytosterols.

Drugs that inhibit prostaglandin synthesis by blocking enzymes that convert arachidonic acid to prostaglandins include aspirin, NSAIDs and acetaminophen. They are responsible for tens of thousands of deaths each year in the states alone. When a respected colleague first discovered this at a major research hospital in the 1960's, he was fired because he wanted to publish the connection he found between NSAIDs and kidney failure, potentially saving more lives than are lost on the highways. The hospital was dependent upon funding from the corporations that manufacture the drugs, so the link was kept under wraps... and still is. In addition to massive over the counter sales of acetylated salicylates (Aspirin, Bayer, Bufferin, and generic), ibuprofen (Advil, Motrin, and generic), and naproxen (Aleve and generic), there are 70 million prescriptions for NSAIDs written for Americans each year. NSAIDs over-alkalize inflamed connective tissues, stopping the body's purposeful detoxification processes by forming a toxic malformed gel out of the toxic sol state that contains whatever toxins the body was trying to eliminate, plus the introduced drug. This turns an acute inflammatory healing response into a chronic, and potentially degenerative disease state, which means a headache suppressed with aspirin is more likely to return again and again as chronic headaches. This is good for the economy.

In contrast, EPA provides a substrate for the anti-aggregatory, anti-inflammatory and vasodilating prostaglandin -3 series. Other effective alternatives for relief of pain and inflammation include a highly absorbable water-soluble quercetin (e.g. Pain Guard Forte' from PerQue).

Studies on omega-3 fatty acid metabolism show:

1. PGE3 and PGD3 lowered intraocular pressure without causing ocular inflammation in rabbit

2. Some surveys demonstrated that in Greenland Eskimos whose marine diet is enriched with omega-3 substrate eicosapentaenoic acid, have a lower incidence of open-angle glaucoma as compared to Caucasians, whose diet is rich in arachidonic acid.The anterior uvea synthesizes PGE3 and PGD3 in human, monkey, and rabbit and may play a role in lowering intraocular pressure. Cyclooxygenase and lipoxygenase pathways in anterior uvea and conjunctiva.

Kulkarni PS, Srinivasan BD. Kentucky Lions Eye Research Institute School of Medicine, University of Louisville 40202. Prog Clin Biol Res 1989; 312: 39-52. Lewith, G., Kenyon, J., Lewis, P. Complementary Medicine: An Integrated Approach 1996, pp. 108-9. New York: Oxford University Press.

Plant sources such as flax seed, hemp seed, chia seed, and walnut provide the precursor Omega-3 fatty acid: Alpha-linolenic acid that the human body converts, though inefficiently, to the longer chain EPA and DHA fatty acids needed for anti-inflammatory prostaglandin formation, neuro-visual development and performance (e.g. DHA for visual acuity) and other cellular needs. Soy and rape-seed (Canola from Canadian Oil Company) also contain ALA but are not recommended as sources by Remission Foundation.

DHA is the #1 fatty acid in the central nervous system. Fish oils contain the Omega-3 fatty acids in their physiologically active EPA and DHA forms for health benefits as immediate PG3 prostaglandin precursors, saving the time and energy of the inefficient enzymatic steps necessary to process Alpha-linolenic acid into the biologically active forms. In many health situations, these enzyme pathways limit the amount of eicosanoids the body can produce to much less than the levels requisite for optimal health and performance.

Nutrients required for the anti-inflammatory EFA pathways to function include:

Essential Fatty Acids (omega-3 and omega-6, in balance)
Zinc
Magnesium
Pyroxidine (vitamin B6) in its active form P5P
Niacin (vitamin B3)
Ascorbic acid (vitamin C)

Enzymes delta-6-desaturase, delta-5-desaturase, elongase, cyclo-oxygenase and oxygenase convert alpha-linolenic acid into the beneficial, anti-inflammatory PGE3 series prostaglandins.

Omega-3 Pathway (Substrate + Enzyme + Cofactors = Product)

Omega-3 EFA substrate + delta-6 desaturase enzyme + B6, Mg, and Zn cofactors = Stearidonic Acid product.

Alpha-linolenic Acid (LNA) substrate + Stearidonic Acid elongase enzyme = Eicosatetraenoic Acid product.

Eicosatetraenoic Acid substrate + delta-5-desaturase enzyme + Vitamin B3, Vitamin C, and Zn cofactors = Eicosapentaenoic Acid (EPA) product.

Eicosapentaenoic Acid (EPA) substrate + cyclo-oxygenase (COX) enzyme = PGE-3. This metabolic pathway is blocked by COX inhibiting drugs.

Eicosapentaenoic Acid (EPA) substrate + Lipoxygenase enzyme = Leukotrienes (less inflammatory). This pathway is promoted by COX inhibiting drugs.

Omega-6 Pathway (Substrate + Enzyme + Cofactors = Product)

Linoleic Acid (LA) substrate + delta-6-desaturase enzyme + B6, Mg, and Zn cofactors = Gamma Linolenic Acid (GLA) product

Gamma Linolenic Acid (GLA) + Gamma Linolenic Acid elongase enzyme = Dihomogamma Linolenic Acid (DGLA)

Dihomogamma Linolenic Acid (DGLA) substrate + delta-5-desaturase enzyme + Vitamin B3, Vitamin C, and Zn cofactors = PGE 1. This is the preferred pathway to anti-inflammatory Series 1 Prostaglandins.

With Omega-3 deficiency

Arachidonic Acid (AA) substrate (prefers Omega-3 oils) + cyclo-oxygenase (COX) enzyme = inflammatory Series 2 Prostaglandins. COX inhibiting drugs block this metabolic pathway involved in the regulation of tissue detoxification.

Several investigators have demonstrated that PGE 2 and PGF 2 alpha in low doses, lower intraocular pressure in all species studied, including human, but while PGF 2 promotes inflammation that could aggravate glaucoma, PGE 2 has anti-inflammatory effects. PGF 2 derivatives are used to medically lower IOP by affecting the FP receptor. These include latanoprost (Xalatan), travoprost (Travatan), bimatoprost (Lumigan) and unoprostone isopropyl (Rescula).

Neurotransmitters

Acetylcholine and seratonin relax the smooth muscle in blood vessels, improving perfusion. This is essential for oxygenation and nutrition, and works in tandem with the movement-activated lymphatic system and the direct current activated meridian systems for tissue detoxification.

Phosphatidyl Choline (PC) is available as a high purity nutritional supplement in capsule form as PhosChol (from Nutracell). PC is used even in intravenous form to dissolve fatty deposits in the blood vessels to improve circulatory perfusion. It also functions as a precursor for the body to make acetylcholine.

The amino acids L-Tryptophan and 5-Hydroxy Tryptophan (5-HTP) are available as nutritional supplements to supply precursors for the body to make seratonin.

For nutritional support for making the catecholamine neurotransmitters, see the next section on amino acids.

Enzymes

Protein deposits in the drainage system of the eye can increase eye pressure by blocking the outflow of fluid from the eye. These proteins that typically accumulate with age may come from inflammatory processes such as allergy, toxicity, radiation and infection, as well as from debris from ocular tissue such as melanin from the iris or exfoliation from the lens. It could also come from partially digested large food proteins such as dairy, wheat, eggs and soy that often cause congestion in the lymphatic system as well. Proteolytic enzymes taken orally may be helpful in breaking down proteins deposited in the trabecular meshwork. This meshwork acts like a filter for the aqueous humor, the fluid, which fills the front of the eye, as the fluid drains out from the eye into a drainage channel called Schlemm's canal. The proteins leak from capillaries in the ciliary body, probably due to inflammation, so other anti-inflammatory therapies may be beneficial in prevention. In addition to proteolytic enzymes like bromelain, papain, trypsin, and chymotrypsin, this may include lipase, amylase, rutin, EPA, L-cysteine or N-acetyl-cysteine, zinc, catalase and SOD. Antioxidant enzymes glutathione peroxidase (dependent on cysteine, selenium and vitamin E) and SOD (dependent on zinc, copper and manganese) have been shown to prevent demyelination of optic nerve fibers caused by the oxidant hydrogen peroxide. Dietary enzymes from raw foods may be beneficial, too. A study in Africa on genetically related tribesmen eating a traditional diet versus those in urban areas with a Western diet, showed less high pressure (a significant risk factor in glaucoma). Traditional diets in general, with less processing and food additives, and containing some raw foods as well as some animal proteins, have been found to be beneficial for prevention of degenerative diseases. Reduced levels of the antioxidant enzymes superoxide dismutase (SOD) and catalase is a risk factor for loss of pigment from the structures inside the eye. This pigment can then clog the drainage channels of the eye leading to pigmentary glaucoma. Rebuilding the antioxidant enzyme levels requires amino acids as well as trace minerals to be available, including adequate copper, zinc, manganese and selenium. While amino acids are important, excessive protein, especially when overcooked or microwaved, and thus more difficult to digest, may be a risk factor for pigmentary glaucoma, especially when dietary protein intake exceeds 3 times the RDA.

Probiotics

Terrain

Friendly flora, like our own eucaryotic cells, are aerobic (oxygen loving). We thrive together in the same terrain. Pathogens, whether bacterial, fungal or parasitic, are typically anaerobic opportunists. They thrive when and where we are not healthy. Just like in a microbiological laboratory, for a particular organism to live and multiply, it must be supplied with a very specific growth medium. A petri dish for growing viruses must contain attenuated cells. The same is true inside the body (in vivo) as it is in a test tube or petri dish (in vitro, meaning in glass). In the 19th century, Bechamp championed this perspective of the terrain, while Pasteur argued for the claim that microbes are causal. In the complex dynamic feedback system that is a living ecosystem such as the human gut, both are necessarily true. So, while Bechamp lost the argument in the 19th century, we must integrate the two claims into a higher order model of health and disease to heal conditions such as glaucoma in the 21st century. Today, we see the limitations of anti-microbial treatment, with the worst infections being nosocomial infections with organisms that have adapted to the demands of the terrain we have modified with fungal toxin analogs (antibiotics), becoming resistant, and in the process, more virulent.

Probiotics

Probiotics are symbiotic microbial flora that enhance the internal mileau of the body. While the bulk of them live in the gut, which is topologically outside the body, they have a tremendous effect on the health of the interior of the body. They produce bulk, enzymes, immune factors and B vitamins. The friendly flora competes with pathogens to keep the body's terrain healthy. To get more benefit from beneficial flora in the upper respiratory tract including the sinuses, in order to benefit the eyes and help improve the terrain in glaucoma, open some of the capsules and take as a powder in the mouth.

In delicate states such as the very elderly, infirm, with young children, or with reactive states such as glaucoma with acute angle closure risk, it is best to start with the gentlest flora, which is the *Bifidobacteria*, sometimes called *Lactobacillus bifidus*. In infants or other very sensitive cases, consider using *Bifidobacteria infantum*. Starting with the smallest dose such as a pinch of powder taken out of a single capsule is the gentlest introduction, which can be followed by ramping the dosage up until a full normal dose is tolerated even by the most sensitive, reactive person. Next, Lactoacidophilus can be added. Then increasingly complete ecosystems composed of greater numbers of species and more aggressive species such as *Streptococcus faecium* can be introduced to leverage ever greater 'sweetening' of the internal terrain of the gut and the eye. The retina has an internal energetic link to the small intestine meridian. This means that the extra-cellular fluid that bathes the retinal cells is directly affected by the health or toxicity present in the tissues of the small intestine.

Soil Based Organisms

Different organisms are able to thrive in different conditions largely because they have different enzymes. Soil Based Organisms (SBOs) are ubiquitous in the natural environments our bodies are designed to thrive in. If your ancestors ate root vegetables, and used their hands for digging and eating, they were constantly exposed to this wide range of organisms. Spontaneous Remission of thousands of cases of cancer documented in the medical literature is always associated with a fever and bacterial overgrowth. Over 200 different species of bacteria have been associated with this natural cure for cancer that only takes a few days! Clinically documented broad spectrum SBOs are available as Prescript Assist from Researched Nutritionals.

Fiber

Prebiotics

Prebiotics are factors that help establish a terrain conducive to the flourishing of symbiotic flora. Prebiotics include oligosaccharide fibers that we cannot digest, but our bacterial helpers can. Beneficial sources include fermented soybeans (tempeh, miso and natto), inulin sources such as Jerusalem artichoke, jicama, and chicory root), raw oats, unrefined barley, and yacon. Also included are fermented foods such as poi, sour kraut, kim chee, miso, tempeh, natto and yogurt. A supplement called SeaCure is based on a traditional fermented white fish protein, and it has remarkable qualities for restoring digestive function especially for those who are underweight and have difficulty gaining enough weight. Along with these prebiotics, other factors which affect the terrain we can provide for our gut flora include eating a diet closer to what our body is genetically adapted to thrive with over millions of years, aspects of which are called the Raw diet, the Paleo diet, or the Blood Type diet. This diet is high in prebiotic fiber with lots of fresh greens, vegetables and also healthy (not commercial) animal or fish protein. Remember, our ancestors ate only organic food!

Chitosan

Based on an 800-year old oriental medicine from Japan, Chitosan (pronounced key-toh-san) is a marine fiber made from chitin, washed alternately with strong acid and alkali solutions. This process removes functional groups, leaving a unique electrically charged fat-soluble fiber that binds strongly to petrochemicals, radioactive minerals and heavy metals. Chitosan works differently than plant fibers because it is fat-soluble and it has the opposite electrical charge of that found on plant fibers. It is used extensively in municipal water treatment, but is also used in medicine for detoxification, weight loss, hypercholesterolemia, cancer and MRSA. By binding bile salts and removing them from the gut before they can be reabsorbed for recycling, Chitosan stimulates the body to mobilize cholesterol from storage on arterial walls in order to use it to make bile in the liver. Lower molecular weight MicroChitosan (made by Allergy Research Group) is available to enhance systemic absorption and detoxification effects.

Botanicals

Coleus forskohlii

Coleus forskohlii is an herb (related to mint) used traditionally in folk medicine in Northern India. It is the only known source of forskolin, a labdane diterpene compound, which activates the enzyme adenylate cyclase, which elevates cAMP, which can then result in a reduction in intraocular pressure (IOP) when applied topically to the eye. Forskolin's unique stimulation of the main catalytic subunit of adenylate cyclase has made it the subject of over 1,000 published scientific studies. Forskolin essentially acts as an amplifier for intracellular communication via the endocrine system. A double-blind study found that a 1% forskolin suspension produced a definite drop in intraocular pressure for 6 hours following use. Another controlled study showed that two instillations of 1% forskolin resulted in a 2.4 mm Hg drop in IOP in just 1 hour, with a 13% reduction in aqueous flow rate. Additional experiments showed that 1% forskolin lowered IOP in humans as well as in rabbits and monkeys, with a drop in outflow pressure of 34 to 70%. Coleus works like Magnesium, by relaxing smooth muscle, plus it has antihistamine properties, perhaps reducing allergic components of increased IOP as well. A dosage of 200 to 400 mg/day of the herb in capsule form has been recommended given the herb's long record of safety. Coleus, for example lowers blood pressure, which often accompanies elevated IOP and is beneficial in asthma and congestive heart failure, conditions, which contraindicate the use of beta-blocker eye drops. Unlike beta-blockers, forskolin enhances ocular blood flow, while having no systemic side effects and not inducing miosis. Those with darker eye color require higher doses than do those with light colored eyes. Synergistic effects can be achieved by combining coleus with omega 6 fatty acids.

How effective is Forskolin at lowering eye pressure?

Here is the example of Dr. Kuakiniokalani Keeaumoku Kawananakoa-Prible, His Serene Highness, Hawaiian Prince and European royalty (he grew up in Buckingham Palace). In his own words, Doctor Kuakini reported to me, "Eye pressure at Hawaiian Eye Clinic: 42 & 46. One month later, eye pressure at Hawaiian Eye Clinic: 30 & 31 without using any eye drops or chemical drugs. Used only herbal caps of Forskohlii." The ophthalmologist at Hawaiian Eye, the #1 eye clinic in Hawaii, had prescribed eye drops, which he had informed Dr. Kuakini he did not expect to work. He was amazed at the reduced eye pressures, thinking that the prescription had worked. When Dr. Kuakini informed him that he had not filled the prescription, since he was told they would not work anyway, but had instead taken an herbal remedy, the ophthalmologist was even more amazed and said that it was the first time he had ever actually seen a natural substance actually reduce a patient's eye pressure.

Ginkgo biloba

Ginkgo biloba was found to actually produce mild improvements in a study on patients with glaucoma and other severe degenerative disorders of the circulation in the back of the eye. This was considered very significant given the very poor prognosis for the conditions treated. Treatment began with 160 mg/day for the first 4 weeks followed by maintenance on 120 mg/day. *Ginkgo biloba* has several biological actions that help against glaucoma:

improves central blood flow including the optic nerve and retina
improves peripheral blood flow
neuroprotection by inhibiting apoptosis

Chung HS, Harris A, Kristinsson JK, Ciulla TA, Kagemann C, Ritch R. Ginkgo biloba extract increases ocular blood flow velocity. J Ocul Pharmacol Ther 1999 Jun;15(3):233-240.Ritch R. Potential role for Ginkgo biloba extract in the treatment of glaucoma. Med Hypotheses 2000; 54: 221-35.In a prospective, randomized, placebo-controlled, double-masked crossover trial at the Glaucoma Center, Clinica Oculistica Universita di Brescia, and the Clinica Oculistica, Universita di Catania, in Italy, GBE improves preexisting visual field damage in some patients with normal tension glaucoma (NTG). 27 patients with bilateral visual field damage resulting from NTG received 40 mg GBE orally three times daily for four weeks, followed by a washout period of eight weeks, and then four weeks of placebo treatment (40 mg fructose). Other patients took the fructose first and the GBE last.

Visual field tests were performed at baseline and the end of each phase of the study. Significant improvements in visual fields indices were found after GBE treatment. Mean deviation (MD) at baseline was 11.40 +/- 3.27 dB versus 8.78 +/- 2.56 dB MD after GBE treatment; corrected pattern standard deviation (CPSD) at baseline was 10.93 +/- 2.12 dB versus 8.13 +/- 2.12 dB CPSD after GBE treatment. No significant changes were found in intraocular pressure (IOP), blood pressure, or heart rate after placebo or GBE treatment. The study concluded that *Ginkgo biloba* extract administration improves preexisting visual field damage in some patients with NTG. Quaranta L, Bettelli S, Uva MG, Semeraro F, Turano R, Gandolfo E. Effect of Ginkgo biloba extract on preexisting visual field damage in normal tension glaucoma. Ophthalmology 2003; 110: 359-62. Some doctors now recommend ginkgo together with vitamin E in glaucoma management. A dosage of 100 to 240 mg/day of ginkgo has been recommended.

Salvia miltiorrhiza

Salvia miltiorrhiza is an herb used traditionally in oriental medicine. A study of patients with middle to late stage glaucoma received a preparation made from the root of this herb for one month. Visual acuity improved in 43.8% of the eyes studied, while 49.7% showed increased visual fields (statistically significant at p<0.01 compared to untreated controls). Followups as long as 30 months continued to show either stable or improved visual fields.

Pilocarpus jaborandi

Pilocarpine is a natural source drug long used to treat glaucoma, being derived from the herb *Pilocarpus jaborandi*. It has also been used in homeopathic doses for this purpose, which is a preferable form especially for people under the age of 40 due to the severe side affects of headaches that often accompany its use in young people.

Cannabis sativa

Research has explored the possible use of the herb *Cannabis sativa* (hemp), either topically on the eye or systemically, to reduce IOP. With the potential to decrease eye pressure by 51%, it is the most effective agent known for IOP reduction. Smoking this herb unfortunately results in numerous side effects including tachycardia (speeding heart rate by 22 to 65%, the opposite of beta-blockers), low blood pressure, a false sense of euphoria, photophobia, blepharospasm, dry eyes, and loss of short-term memory. Extracts of this herb were used widely in medicine until early in this century. Now, hemp oil is becoming available, and is an excellent source of essential fatty acids to nourish the nerves of the eye. Tinctures and homeopathics, however, remain unavailable. The herb has been banned even for medical purposes since 1992.

Vaccinium myrtillus

Bilberry (*Vaccinium myrtillus*), taken at a dosage equivalent to 1/4 teaspoon of solid extract 3 times a day has been recommended for all types of glaucoma. This herb has been shown to improve visual function in a variety of conditions including myopia, night blindness and diabetic retinopathy. The blue-red pigments (anthocyanosides) found in this and other berries have been show to improve vitamin C utilization, improve capillary integrity, provide anti-oxidant protection and stabilize the collagen matrix by directly cross-linking with collagen and preventing enzymatic breakdown of this backbone of the connective tissue.

Zingiber officinalis

Ginger (*Zingiber officinalis*) stimulates improve heart function and increased circulation. A dosage of 100 mg/day of ginger has been recommended.

Capsicum

Capsaicin cream (from cayenne pepper: *Capsicum*) increases circulation in the choroid of the eye, as does electrical stimulation of the trigeminal nerve. Capsicum capsules can also be taken internally, reducing cholesterol, providing antioxidant activity, relaxing smooth muscle for vasodilation and improved circulation, as well as stimulating digestive functions for better nutrient assimilation.

Allium sativum

Garlic (*Allium sativum*), which improves circulation, blood pressure and cholesterol levels, while providing antioxidant properties, has been recommended at a dosage of 500 to 1000 mg/day.

Crataegus oxyacantha

Hawthorne berries have been suggested to improve heart rhythm and thus enhance circulation, while lowering hypertension and cholesterol where such cardiovascular problems are present together with glaucoma.

Spirulina pacifica

Spirulina has been reported to help restore vision lost due to glaucoma.

Glycerin

Vegetable source glycerin (1 to 2 g/kg body weight) mixed with an equal amount of water or juice can be used for first aid in acute angle closure glaucoma attacks.

Eyewash & Eye drops

Several herbs may be combined or alternated as a warm eyewash or in eye drop form (3 drops in each eye, instilled 3 times a day), including *Coleus forskohlii*, fennel, chamomile and eyebright.

Homeopathy

Homeopathic Medicines

Several practitioners have written about their success in treating glaucoma with homeopathic remedies. Remedies in itallics are more frequently found useful. Descriptions in italics are key symptoms in confirming the selection of the remedy.

Aconite: at beginning of acute attack with much heat, redness and burning pain in eye, together with fever.

Asafoetida: severe boring pain over the eye and around it.

Aurum metallicum: glaucoma with tendency toward blindness, upper half of objects invisible, with atherosclerosis and suicidal depression.

Belladonna: severe glaucoma pain with throbbing headache and flushed face; eyes injected, pupils dilated, fundus hyperemic with pain in and around eye; pains may come and go suddenly, worse in afternoon and evening; eyes hot and dry with light sensitivity; reddish halo around lights.

Bryonia: useful in early stages of acute glaucoma attacks; eyes feel full as if pressed out, often with sharp, shooting pains through the eye and head. The eyes feel sore to the touch and on moving them in any direction. Halo around lights, with heavy pain over eye, worse at night.

Cedron: severe shooting pains along the supraorbital nerve.

Colocynthus: severe, burning, aching, sticking or cutting pains in and around eye, relieved by firm pressure and by walking in a warm room; aggravated by rest at night and on stooping.

Gelsemium: very frequently useful clinically in glaucoma with heavy eyelids (ptosis), dim vision, one or both pupils fixed and dilated, pain and twitching of muscles, bruised pain behind eyes, with dizziness, drowsiness, dullness and trembling or muscle weakness or paralysis. Patient may not seem to care about his condition.

Nux vomica: marked morning aggravation; atrophy of optic nerve due to glaucoma.

Osmium: sudden, sharp severe pains in and around eye; dim, foggy vision; halo with colors around lights.

Phosphorus applies to inflamed nerves and hemorrhages that suddenly destroy nerve cells. The eyes fatigue easily. Green halos may be seen around lights and letters may appear red. Optic atrophy is also typical. The conjunctiva appears pearly white but there may be swelling of the eyelids.

Prunus spinosa: severe, crushing pain in eye, as if the eye were pressed asunder, or sharp pain shooting through the eye and same side of the head (similar to Spigelia); hazy aqueous and vitreous; fundus hyperemic.

Rhododendron: incipient glaucoma, with alot of pain periodically in and around eye, always worse just before a storm and better once the storm begins.

Spigelia: sharp, stabbing pains through the eye and head, worse with motion and worse at night.

Other individual remedies to consider include Arnica, Arsenicum, Atrop., Causticum, Chamomilla, Cocaine (homeopathic not available in the states even in potencies with no chemical coca content), Commocl., Conium, Croc., Croton tiglium, Eser., Hamamelis, Kali iodatum, Macrotin., Mag. carb., Mercurius, Op. (not available in the states), Pilocarpus, Rhus toxicodendron, and Sulfur.

Other commonly used remedies for retrobulbar neuritis include Arsenicum album, Nux vomica and Terebenthina, while less frequently prescribed homeopathics are Ferrum phosphoricum and Kali phosphoricum.

Optic atrophy is treated by Argentum nitricum, Arsenicum album, Nux vomica, especially if alcohol, tobacco or other drugs are used, Phosphorus, Plumbum metallicum, with small pupils and inflammation of the optic nerve (as in multiple sclerosis), Strychninum phosphoricum, Veratrum viride (American hellebore), Zincum phosphoricum.

Complex Homeopathy

Many practitioners also recommend complex homeopathy for lymphatic drainage and treatment of underlying energetic causes of glaucoma. Excellent remedies include Lymphomyosot (from BHI) for lymphatic drainage support, and some of the author's formulas: Energessence (for lymphatic and blood circulation, oxygenation), Stamina Plus (for stress), Food Tolerance (for food allergy) and AllerFree (for airborne allergies) to balance underlying causal factors. Homeopathic Proteolytic Enzymes (e.g. Digestzymes), vitamins and minerals (e.g. Natural Resource A-Z) may also be used.

Sarcodes

Sarcodes are homeopathic remedies made from healthy tissue. Relevant sarcodes for electrodermal testing and potentially for homeopathic treatment include adrenal (Supraren ext.), heart-related sarcodes, carotid artery, lymph node, the eye (Oculus totalis), ciliary body, aqueous humor, Schlemm's canal, retina, optic nerve, lamina cribrosa and Chromosome 1. Purified extracts of healthy tissues, such as homeopathic cholesterol (steroidal hormone precursor), pregnenolone, progesterone, estrogen, epinephrine, melatonin,

GABA, seratonin, acetylcholine, DHEA and 7-Keto DHEA are also potentially useful for both diagnosis and treatment.

Nosodes

Nosodes are homeopathic preparations made from diseased tissues, such as pseudoexfoliation or pigmentary dispersion.

The nosode Brucella abortus Bang can affect the eye and optic nerve area, including in MS and glaucoma.

So-called imponderable homeopathics, such as IOP, and including nosodes such as 60 Hz can be used diagnostically and therapeutically.

Homeopathics of herbs and allopathic medications may also be used.

Autonosodes are made from the patient's own body, such as blood (autohemonosode) or urine (homeopathic can be free of any taste that might be an issue for many to try 'water of life' therapy) to stimulate the homeostatic regulatory processes including recruiting additional detoxification pathways. Technically, this is a form of isopathy (iso means same, versus homeo meaning similar).

In addition, the following remedies may be useful, as they are known to cause the condition in toxic doses: Amyl alcohol (methanol), Atoxyl, Cannabis indicus (hashish, not available in the states as a homeopathic remedy), Carbon bisulphide, Dinitrobenzol, Iodoformium,

Nitrobenzol, Plumbum (lead, Pb), Stramonium (jimson weed) and Tabacum (tobacco).

Color, Light and EMF

Ultraviolet Light

Ultraviolet protective eyewear is frequently recommended to reduce photo-oxidative stress in the eye. Even UV absorbing contact lenses are now available. This may help reduce oxidative stress on ocular tissues and reduce the risk of exfoliation of lens proteins that can clog the trabecular meshwork. Exfoliation is seen more in people who spend more time outdoors and in sunnier environments. The same people show changes in the eyelids, and excessive sunlight is known to reduce the elasticity of connective tissues. It appears to be UV-B radiation (280-320 nanometers) that damages the lens cells that exfoliate, although antioxidants are known to protect against this damage.

Visible Light Frequencies

Wearing green glasses may be helpful. Typically, cool colors such as blue-green, blue, indigo and violet are used directly in the eyes in glaucoma, since these stimulate the parasympathetic nervous system, contracting the pupil to increase drainage of the aqueous humor and reduce IOP. Syntonic phototherapy using color stimulation of the retina has been shown to increase visual fields in a number of studies in various populations. Both fluorescent and incandescent artificial lights are deficient in these cool colors, resulting in chronic stress, and contributing to glaucoma as well as 85% of all disease. Full spectrum lighting provides a more natural indoor light which reduces systemic and eye stress, while improving calcium metabolism. Full spectrum light reduces hip fractures by 50%, while medical treatment for glaucoma has been shown to increase hip fractures by over 300%. This point is especially important not because medical treatment for hip fracture costs $25,000 per patient, but because one third of these patients will die within one year following a fractured hip.

For treating the whole body with light, Dinshah recommends yellow-green on the entire front of the body, followed by indigo on the eyes, and magenta on the heart and kidney areas.

EMF

Electromagnetic Fields are an important issue in chronic degenerative diseases like glaucoma, because one third of patients do not respond to a comprehensive, well tailored remedial program until interference from natural or technical electromagnetic fields are eliminated as a block to cure. While the basics of resolving these issues are covered in the book Electromagnetic Pollution Solutions, the retina is particularly sensitive as its design function is to be an electromagnetic receptor. The most crucial steps are to eliminate electronic devices and their power cords from around the bed, since the body is most sensitive while sleeping, and attempting to cleanse and regenerate. Therapeutically, grounding the body by a barefoot walk on the beach or on unsprayed grass, or even a shower with the drain plugged and some epsom salts or sea salt to increase conductivity to connect the body to the earth helps to restore the body's supply of free electrons, the ultimate anti-oxidant.

Acupuncture & Electro-Acupuncture

Acupuncture can help otherwise incurable eye diseases. Enkephalin, which is released in acupuncture, reduces IOP. Acupuncture may be able to slow progressive vision loss when drugs can't. Acupuncture may also be able to help reverse optic atrophy. Acupuncture together with Vitamin B12 was able to control glaucoma in a dog. Acupuncture is synergistic with homeopathy and other forms of natural medicine.

Electrodermal Screening

Electrodiagnostic modalities like Electroacupuncture According to Voll (EAV), the Vegetative Reflex Test (VRT, formerly called the Vegatest Method) of Schimmel or other functional testing methods are often used to determine the optimum therapy, including homeopathy as well as nutrition, and even pharmaceuticals. Such methods of European Diagnostic Electroacupuncture are also termed Electrodermal Screening (EDS).

In the EAV system, there are points around the bony rim of the orbit of each eye that link electronically to various parts of the eye. In glaucoma, the most important points typically include measurement points for the frontal sinus, the sclera, the retina, the choroid, the vitreous body, the ciliary body, and the iris as well as the summation measurement points for the anterior and posterior segments of the eye.

High impedence measurements above 65 indicate inflammatory tendency in the associated tissue. Low measurements below 50 indicate chronic degenerative tendency. Any unsustained measurements, referred to as an indicator drop, indicate the presence in that extracellular fluid channel of incompletely ionizing toxins.

Measurements are observed to normalize to within the clinically normal range of 50 to 65 with sustainability essentially instantaneously when a well-suited (energetically resonant) medicine is brought within the body's biofield. As seen on Kirlian high voltage imagery, this field extends approximately 1 centimeter from the body's biological tissue. German studies have confirmed that the response is to radiant energy, as the response remains robust through a vacuum of up to 1 centimeter.

In practice, these eye points are often challenging but not impossible (with an armamentarium of many hundreds of potential natural medicines) to bring to balance, especially when readings show intense and widespread inflammatory energy. As a foundational support for accelerated self-healing, I always balance the control measurement points (CMP) for all the major vessels on both hands and both feet before attempting to balance the eye points.

Once a coherent systemic and ocular state of energetic balance is accomplished the first time, subsequent balancing is usually significantly easier and simpler to restore. This can be done as often as necessary, typically every other week, for a few sessions, with the tested home OTC remedies being used between sessions to support the accelerated self-healing that results from all major body systems working in a balanced and coherent state. Once a degree of stability is achieved, I find that monthly adjustment of remedies is ideal. Only when full health is restored is a more lax seasonal balancing recommended, since the acceleration of the body's natural cleansing and healing mechanisms result in completion of incomplete healing and detoxification responses, leading to the potential for healing reactions as older and deeper layers are retraced.

The same points can be used for self-healing by massaging in a gentle circular motion. Only comfortable fingertip pressure should be used, focusing on healing intent and receptivity to feeling the flow of healing energy from the fingers to the parts of the eye, and with openness to feeling any internal energy shifts within the eye and body.

Remote biocommunication, developed through many years of electrodermal practice with Dr. Helmut Schimmel's Vegatest Method, and adapted to utilize the sensitivity developed with modification of Dr. Omura's O-Ring method has also provided a means of effective surrogate energetic evaluation and analysis at a distance. While electronic point measurement often provides inroads to greater depth and detail of information in the body's energetic compensatory system, the accuracy and effectiveness of surrogate and remote kinesiological and other subtle subjective methods of biofeedback can become fully as accurate and coherent with the information obtained by the technical means. In practice, after years of utilizing a variety of approaches, I prefer, when working in person, to observe both views. This offers a kind of 'stereoscopic' view of the energetic responses, with the first being the more subjective and subtle, so that there is less data to potentially influence the more sensitive testing. This can rapidly and efficiently provide an average of about 80% of the remedy identification information needed to balance all 40 CMP points of the Bioelectronic Functions Diagnosis (BFD) method, which I use to confirm and extend the initial subjective observations.

Outro

Standard management of glaucoma is primarily suppressive in effect. Suppression of symptomatic body functions tends to impair the body's completion of its corrective response to the initiating cause, and thus to prolong the pathophysiological state, adding an iatrogenic layer to the pathogenesis.

Natural medicines that modulate immune function (such as phytosterols), may be compatible with the suppressed state, as they reduce the inflammatory responses in allergy, which is associated with glaucoma, while they increase immunity against infectious agents.

When fundamental biophysical parameters of internal mileau/terrain are restored toward normal and thus toward a more coherent state, the physiological patterns change periodically (lunar biorhythmic condensate cycle) in the varied course of healing processes, which must of necessity include a degree of freedom for the immune system to activate its oxidative, inflammatory and thermogenic pathways, as these are essential in the process of tissue cleansing, which must precede fully functional repair of impaired tissue.

Bio-energetic Regulatory Status is typically quite low in glaucoma, I believe in large part because of the suppressive chemistry of the beta-adrenergic receptor blockers. This means that some of the body's normal functional responses are blocked. Suppressive therapies such as antibiotics and other anti-inflammatories, including adrenal corticosteroids (but not including the safer OTC steroids such as 7-Keto DHEA) intensely and prematurely alkalize tissue solubilized for restoration of a clean fresh connective tissue matrix, which serves as the filter through which processes of nutrition, elimination and biocommunication must flow. Recent findings with cancer cells are illustrative for other chronic degenerative diseases, such as most glaucomas, which are caused proximally by pathophysiological patterns seen in Phase 1, Low Energy Terrain, in which only 10% of the normal cellular energy production is functional, that being the fermentation pathways of the cytoplasm, lacking the aerobic mitochondrial function, whether that symbiosis is impaired primarily by tissue hypoxia related to a local or systemic reduction in oxygenation and/or perfusion. A non-chlorine based oxygen catalyst (Cell Food, Cell Renew or Cell Silver) is a favorite natural remedy to test for such a situation, as it is designed to raise the partial pressure of oxygen. This can begin to reduce the backlog of lactic acid in the tissue that sustains the ischemic condition. Eliminating EMF from the sleeping area is essential for allowing the EKG signal to open the arterioles, necessary for 50% of optimal tissue oxygenation. Supplying free electrons not only provides a first line antioxidant defense against on of the final common pathways of tissue damage, aging and degenerative disease, along with processes of glycation (forming AGE, Advanced Glycation

Endproducts), cross-linking of fibers, constricting the connective tissue matrix

Afterword

The author was a 25-year old interning eye doctor at the world's largest outpatient vision clinic in New York City, and president of the American Optometric Student Association, representing over 4000 student doctors of optometry worldwide when he learned that he had glaucoma. Knowing that the best medical and surgical treatment would likely leave him blind before age 50, he embarked on his continuing investigation of alternative, complementary, and integrative medical approaches to the treatment, prevention and rehabilitation of glaucoma and other eye and vision conditions. 30 years later, he continues to maintain his vision without suppressive eye drops or invasive eye surgery.

Conclusion

Much opportunity lies ahead in natural medicine for healing the various forms and underlying causes of glaucoma. The most important element, in my estimation, is to further the development of our science in support of a modern art of healing in which the unique response characteristics of each individual can be observed in real time. Science is fundamentally observation. When any treatment is instituted blind, that is without some probe of the treated systems response prior to full clinical trial, we are operating in a realm of trial and error. The current state of the art in evidence based medicine rests mostly on extrapolation from population based evidence. Unfortunately, it is also frequently skewed and incomplete evidence even at the population level due to financial incentives in the corporate world of pharmaceutical commerce, the most lucrative industry in the world. Most negative data is suppressed. Some positive data is even falsified. Economic incentives favor patent medicines and surgical procedures, both of which almost invariably start with transgression of the physician's sacred oath to first do no harm, since most drugs have side effects and surgery is controlled damage by definition.

When a patient presents a family history of glaucoma, or signs of being a glaucoma suspect... even when there is a borderline expression of glaucomatous signs, or an early stage of open angle glaucoma, there is a window of opportunity to explore the vast and largely uncharted territory of accelerated self healing.

Once suppressive drug therapy has begun, a course is set, the natural history of which is not attractive, and intercurrent therapies with natural medicine, especially for detoxification of heavy metals and other neurotoxins such as pesticides becomes much more fraught with challenge, due to the conflicting purposes of medication aimed largely at suppression of fluid circulation through the anterior chamber of the eye, versus the body's attempts to flush toxins out of that same eye, a process which by its nature involves a temporary conversion of gel to sol state with an accumulation of protons (acidity) and water (reflected in the eye as an elevation in IOP) in the affected connective tissue.

Like the kidneys, the eyes are wrapped tightly with connective tissue, the sclera in the case of the eye, and so a degree of finesse and gentleness is commended in supporting the challenge of cleansing and regenerating such constrained organ tissues as the eye's sensitive nerve fibers as they pass through the lamina cribrosa.

Postscript

When I think back on my life, and realize what different choices I could have made along the way... the most profound paths I have walked have been the ones "less traveled by..."

When I learned at age 26 that I would most likely be blinded by glaucoma well before my present age if I took the conventional approach to managing the disease, I chose to explore all the unconventional approaches to seek a better outcome.

Now, 30 years later, my visual fields are as full as they were then. My intraocular pressures are considerably lower than they were then, achieved without a single prescription drug.

That is not to say that this path has always been easy, or without its own challenges... I have endured massive amounts of dental restoration work to eliminate the source of heavy metals from my teeth, just a few centimeters from the eyes. I have experienced countless symptoms as my body cleared the bioaccumulation of toxins from various tissues, all in its own sequence and timing... but with support. Support from a means of communication, centered on listening to the active response patterns of the body, and noticing when the introduction of a potential therapeutic energy resulted in a quieting, a dampening of any of those active stress responses engaged in by the body's remarkable intelligence, an intelligence that is founded in the eons of the past, of surviving, of healing, of cleansing and repairing with only what nature had to offer... only the tens of thousands of biological remedies our bodies are made to live and work and heal with in the natural environment. Natural medicine is an ongoing exploration with eons of successful research behind it. Modern pharmaceuticals by comparison, are not even a tick of the second hand... a brief experiment, and one governed not by the biological intelligence that processes billions of bits every second, or even by the sensory awareness (mostly visual) of some 10 million bits per second, but by the rational mind, limited as it is to sequential processing on the order of 100 bits per second.

Glossary

AGE: Advanced Glycation Endproducts are the damaging result of excess sugars binding to the body's tissues.

Anti-oxidant: by definition this is an electron donor. The most efficient source of electrons is to ensure we are connected to them from the earth, and are supplying them in abundance in the air and water. This preserves nutritional anti-oxidants for their important co-enzyme functions.

Avascular: lacking a direct blood supply. The interior tissues of the eye, and even the macula lutea in the central retina, in order to be optically clear lack blood vessels once the tissue develops in utero. The remnants of the hyaline artery, active during gestation, cast shadows on the retina, called muscae voluntantes (physiological floaters).

Brunescent: a yellowing of the crystalline lens of the eye.

BEV: see Bio-electronics of Vincent

Bio-Electronics of Vincent (BEV):BEV is an objective means of measuring and calculating energy based on both the electrical (electron) and magnetic (proton) factors in addition to the energetic information factor (photon) via ion content or conductivity (the inverse of resistivity). BEV measurement and analysis can be applied to blood, urine, saliva, water, nutrients, or other substances via measurement of the standard physical parameters: pH, rH2 or O.R.P., and resistivity.

Biokinesiology:Biokinesiology is an advanced method of muscle testing which integrates biocommunication protocols from European electro-dermal testing (see Vegetative Reflex Test and Electroacupuncture According to Voll).

Cataract: a loss of clarity of the crystalline lens of the eye. Clarity of the lens is one of the best known predictors of longevity.

Carrier frequency:A carrier frequency is the frequency or rate at which an oscillating pattern repeats. It acts as the carrier of the information contained in the characteristic pattern of the waveform. The carrier determines the energy content of the individual photons, which transmit the wave. Each specific carrier frequency is like a different AM (amplitude modulation) radio station.

Characteristic waveform: The characteristic waveform is the shape of an electromagnetic oscillation. It is determined by its specific source and represents information content of the electromagnetic oscillation. A characteristic waveform is like the programming on a radio station.

Ciliary Body: the nearest circulation to the lens of the eye, and thus its remote source of nutrition. Like the joints, the lens itself is an avascular tissue.

Crystalline Lens: the lens in the eye that is the densest protein in the body, the most exposed tissue to ionizing radiation, and particularly sensitive to oxidation by free radicals and glycation by sugars (producing AGE), two of the dominant processes of unhealthy aging.

Dowsing: Dowsing is an ancient art of finding water or other substances through amplification of subtle body responses. Dowsers may use wooden or metal dowsing rods, a pendulum, radionic instruments or other convenient amplification devices.

Dry Eye Syndrome: Most often a lack of mucin, the protein which makes the cornea wettable. This is stimulated by Vitamin A, which can be supplied directly in the form of eye drops. More severe cases often involve metal toxicity as well.

Dysbiosis: an imbalance in the normal flora of the body. The body is not a sterile monoculture, but a symbiotic polyculture, right down to the mitochondria, an intracellular bacterium inherited exclusively through the maternal line.

Electroacupuncture According to Voll:EAV is a form of electrodermal remedy testing developed in 1953 by Rheinhold Voll, a German dentist and medical doctor. This system allows the measurement of points and meridians that correspond to specific internal body organs and functions.

Electromagnetic: Electromagnetic field radiation is composed of electrical, magnetic and information components. Electrostatic fields are produced by stationary electrical charges, such as the capacitor in a television set (even when unplugged). Magnetic fields are produced by electrical charges in constant motion, as in a direct current. When electrical charges change their pattern of motion, as in alternating current, electromagnetic radiation is produced. Information is carried in carrier and characteristics waveforms as well as scalar (information only) waves.

Electronic factor: The concentration of electrons in a fluid medium, such as in all biological systems is one of 3 factors, which determine biological energy via the Nernst equation. The other two factors are the magnetic factor and the ion content (electrical conductivity). Because free electrons quickly combine with free protons to produce hydrogen (H2), their concentration is measured as a function of hydrogen molecules (rH2).

Fovea Centralis: normally the point of maximum visual clarity, except in night vision, since there are no rod cells in the macular area.

Glaucoma: Wrongly defined as high pressure in the eyes (IOP) even by most physicians, since a high percentage of glaucomatous eyes actually have low pressure. Glaucoma has many patterns related to nutritional deficiencies and toxicities, but is ultimately the result of damage to the optic nerve.

Healing Crisis: this can be a flu-like reaction observed when taking a stimulatory medicine such as homeopathy. It can be based in a cleansing or detoxification reaction, eliminating stored toxins, or can be a Herxheimer, or die-off process, eliminating bacterial endotoxins or other wastes in the case of dysbiosis.

Hertz: The number of oscillations per second of an electromagnetic field is given the unit Hertz (Hz).

Homeopathy: Homeopathic substances are produced by successive dilution and succussion, resulting in increasing potencies containing increasing electromagnetic carrier frequencies and decreasing chemical concentrations.

Homotoxicology: Homotoxicology is the study of toxins in man. As toxins penetrate further into the system, they may enter more vital organs and tissues. They may also interfere at deeper levels within the cell and ultimately the nucleus. The reversal of this process is marked by a shift in symptoms to more superficial or less vital areas according to anatomy and histology. This detoxification process may also be marked by local metabolism of toxins accompanied inflammatory symptoms, and by increased elimination through mucus membranes, skin, urine or feces.

Homeopathy: the leading form of medicine in the world today in terms of numbers of people treated, and a non-toxic medicine, free of side effects, that works by hormesis, stimulating the body to heal itself by recruiting pathways of response that have been dormant, often due to adaptation to past stresses. Modern science is finally catching up with the field of epigenetics. For over 200 years doctors in this field have watched the non-genetic inheritance of miasms.

Hormesis: The law of dosage effect in pharmacology, also known as the Arndt-Schultz law. Small doses stimulate the body's healing mechanisms. Moderate doses irritate and suppress the ability of those pathways to produce a functional response. Larger doses destroy the same cells.

Ion: A positively or negatively charged particle is an ion. Ions are capable of carrying electrical energy within the body by their movement. The total ion concentration determines the electrical conductivity of a fluid, which is one of 3 factors determining the total energy content according to the Nernst equation. The other two are the electrical and the magnetic factors.

IOP: Intra-Ocular Pressure. High pressure is always an issue, but low or normal pressure does not guarantee health eye tissues and good visual function.

Macula Lutea: the yellow spot in the center of the retina is avascular tissue at the center of which is the Fovea Centralis, normally the point of maximum visual clarity, except in night vision, since their are no rod cells in the macula. The macula has the highest oxygen demand of any tissue in the body, and is energetically linked to the lungs.

Magnetic factor: The concentration of protons, which are positively charged ions, is measured by the magnetic factor (pH). It is one of the 3 basic factors, which determine the amount of biological energy via the Nernst equation. The other factors are the electrical factor and the ion content or electrical conductivity.

Mitochondria: supply 90% of the healthy cell's energy through aerobic metabolism via the electron transport chain, which relies on the B Vitamins as co-factors, and on Oxygen to receive the spent electrons once energy has been extracted for storage and use as ATP.

Muscae Voluntantes: The remnants of the hyaline artery, active during gestation, cast shadows on the retina, as physiological floaters. Toxins in the colon and food reactions can make this shadow darker and more annoying.

Multi-dimensional: Multi-dimensional refers to any process, which has more than just one or two dimensions or key factors. In truth, everything is multi-dimensional. It is only our limited perception, representation or thinking about something that can appear linear (1D) or flat (2D). Space is multi-dimensional (3D). Space-time, which Einstein conceived to be inseparable except by the perception of each individual observer, is 4D. Physicists may now view the universe as 6D, l0D or 26D depending on the context and model proposed.

Pendulum:A pendulum is a simple device consisting of a suspended weight used to amplify subtle neuromuscular patterns in the arm for the detection of biological responses to subtle electromagnetic energy fields.

PSC: Posterior Subcapsular Cataract. This is often a fast onset cataract affecting younger people than most other types. It often relates to immune function and typically responds very well to certain remedies including TMG and Cernilton Flower Pollen.

Radiesthesia:Radionics is an approach to detection of biological responses to subtle electromagnetic energy fields using a stick-plate, which is rubbed by the fingertips. Amplification of subtle physiological changes takes place via noticeable changes in the feel and sound of the stickiness of the stick-plate. Numbers called rates may be used to identify various fields, just as these fields might be identified by names or by numbers such as frequencies, wavelengths, or other characteristics of an electromagnetic oscillation.

Retracing: the tendency to reverse the steps of disease, only much faster in most cases, in the course of the healing process.

Soil Based Organisms (SBO): providing enzyme systems for detoxification, biological transmutation of elements and other functions to assist in altering the course of chronic health issues.

Spectroscopy:A spectroscope measures the intensity of different frequencies of electromagnetic radiation. It is not able to measure the characteristic waveforms of the radiation. The information provided by spectroscopy is therefore like knowing what channels are on the air, but not being able to identify the programming. The most sensitive indicators of the characteristic information in electromagnetic radiation are the physiological responses of biological systems.

Strabismus: an eye that turns in a different direction than its fellow eye. Typically eyes turn in with an increase in acidity that causes increased muscle tension in the extra-ocular muscles, since the Medial Rectus muscles have the largest cross sectional diameter. When the metabolism becomes blocked by an even larger accumulation of the toxin, the pH swings to alkaline, and muscle tone drops below normal, resulting in an outward eye turn. In the course of restoring healthy function, it is often observed that the outward tendency (exo) will convert to inward (eso) on its way to restoring balance. This reversal of the pathway of disease in the healing process is called the eso-exo swing in this context, and in general is a form of retracing.

Vegatetative Reflex Test: Formerly called the Vegatest Method, developed in 1979 by Dr. . Helmut Schimmel, this is a method of electronic monitoring of skin resistance at an acupuncture point. Homeopathic stimuli are used to determine the patterns of causality and relief from stress at that time.

Healing Glaucoma

Vincent: see Bio-electronics of Vincent

Vitreous Body: the jelly like substance filling the back part of the eye, behind the lens. This is where most floaters occur. The vitreous is energetically linked to the large intestine.

Bibliography

Alternative Medicine: The Definitive Guide (Compiled by The Burton Goldberg Group, Future Medicine Publishing, Inc., Puyallup, Washington, 1993).

Balch JF and Balch PA. Prescription for Nutritional Healing. Garden City Park, NY: Avery Publishing Group, 1990.

Berridge EW. Diseases of the Eyes. Jain Publishers, New Delhi, 1984.

Brinker F. Herb Contraindications and Drug Interactions (Eclectic Medical Publications, Sandy, Oregon, 1998).

Burr HS. Blueprint for Immortality: The Electric Patterns of Life (C.W. Daniel Co. Ltd., Saffron Walden, England, 1972).

Chidre D, and Martin H with Beech D. The Heartmath Solution (HarperSanFrancisco, 1999).

Deville M. The Real Trace Element Problem: Their Therapeutic Applications (Centre de Recherches et d'Applications sur les Oligo-Elements).

Dinshah D. Let There Be Light (Dinshah Health Society, Malaga, New Jersey, 1985).

Gerber R. Vibrational Medicine: New Choices for Healing Ourselves (Bear & Company, Santa Fe, New Mexico, 1988).

Grossman, M and Swartwout G. Natural Eye Care, An Encyclopedia: Complementary Treatments for Improving and Saving Your Eyes (Keats Publishing, Los Angeles, 1999).

Hahnemann, S. Organon of Medicine (J.P. Tarcher, Inc., Los Angeles, 1982, translated from original written by Samuel Hahnemann 1755—1843.

Hollwich, F. The Influence of Ocular Light Perception on Metabolism in Man and in Animal (Springer Verlag, New York, Heidelberg, Berlin, 1979).

Jackson M and Teague T. The Handbook of Alternatives to Chemical Medicine. (Oakland, California: Teague and Jackson, 1985)

Kappel G. Nutrition and Vision, OEP Foundation, Santa Ana, Calif. 1980.

Kavner RS and Dusky L. Total Vision, (AW Visual Library, New York, 1978).

Kenyon, JN. Modern Techniques of Acupuncture: A Scientific Guide to Bioelectronic Regulatory Techniques and Complex Homeopathy (Thorsons Publishing Group, Wellingborough, England, 1985).

Kervran CL. Biological Transmutations (Beekman Publishers, Inc., New York, 1971; originally published in French by L Courrier du Livre, 1966).

Kutsky RJ. Handbook of Vitamins, Minerals and Hormones (Van Nostrand Reinhold Company, New York, 1981).

Lane B. Nutrition and Vision, 273-274, in Bland J, Ed. 1984-85 Yearbook of Nutritional Medicine (New Canaan, Connecticut: Keats, 1985).

Mandel P. Energy Emission Analysis: New Applications of Kirlian Photography for Holistic Health (Synthesis, W Germany)

Mandel P. Practical Compendium of Colorpuncture (Energetik Verlag, Bruchsal, W Germany, 1986).

Manning CA and Vanrenen LJ. Bioenergetic Medicines East and West: Acupuncture and Homeopathy (North Atlantic Books, Berkeley, California 1988).

Moffat JL. Homoeopathic Therapeutics in Ophthalmology. Jain Publishers, New Delhi, 1982.

Murphy R. Homeopathic Medical Repertory: A Modern Alphabetic Repertory (Hahnemann Academy of North America, 1993).

Norton AB. Ophthalmic Diseases and Therapeutics. Jain Publishers, New Delhi, 1987.

Ober C, Sinatra ST, and Zucker M.   Earthing: The most important health discovery ever? (Basic Health Publications, Inc., Laguna Beach, California, 2010).

Oschman JL.   Energy Medicine: The Scientific Basis (Churchill Livingstone, an imprint of Harcourt Publishers Ltd, 2000).

Page LR. Healthy Healing. (Sacramento, California: Spilman Printing, 1990)

Pearson D and Shaw S.   Life Extension, A practical scientific approach, (Warner Books, New York, 1983).

Pischinger A.   Matrix and Matrix Regulation: Basis for a Holistic Theory in Medicine (Haug International, Brussels, 1991, 1st German edition 1975).

Pizzorno JE and Murray MT.   A Textbook of Natural Medicine. Seattle, WA: John Bastyr College Publications, 1987.

Randolph TG and Moss RW.   An Alternative Approach to Allergies (Bantam Books, New York, 1980).

Sardi B.   Nutrition and the Eyes.   (Montclair, California: Health Spectrum Publishers, 1994)

Shils ME, Olson JA and Shike M.   Modern Nutrition in Health and Disease, Eighth Edition (Williams & Wilkins, Media, PA, 1994).

Smith CW and Best S. Electromagnetic Man (St. Martin's Press, New York, 1989).

Spitler HR. The Syntonic Principle: Its Relation to Health and Ocular Problems (College of Syntonic Optometry, Eaton, Ohia, 1941).

Stortebecker P. Dental Caries as a Cause of Nervous Disorders (Stortebecker Foundation for Research, Stockholm, Sweden, 1982).

Stortebecker P. Mercury Poisoning from Dental Amalgam - A Hazard to Human Brain (Stortebecker Foundation for Research, Stockholm, Sweden, 1985).

Swartwout GM. Biofields: The New Physics of Health.

Swartwout GM. Electromagnetic Pollution Solutions: What You Can Do To Keep Your Home and Workplace Safe.

Swartwout GM. Glaucoma Solutions: Prevention and Reversal.

Swartwout GM. Vision for Living, 1983.

Swartwout GM. Refreshing Vision: Opening the Windows of the Soul

Swartwout GM. Healing Glaucoma

Swartwout GM. Cataract Solutions: Prevention & Reversal Via Accelerated Self-Healing

Swartwout GM. Macular Degeneration... ...Macular Regeneration

Swartwout GM. The Shire: Glendalf's Guide to Cultivating Your Future Self

Swartwout GM. Materia Medica: Vis Medicatrix Naturae

Swartwout GM. Nous Energy: Healing Power of the Pyramids

Todd GP. Nutrition, Health & Disease. Norfolk, Virginia: Donning Co., 1985.

Valnet J. The Practice of Aromatherapy: A Classic Compendium of Plant Medicines &Their Healing Properties (Healing Arts Press, Rochester, Vermont, 1980, English translation 1982).

Voll R. 2nd Supplement to the Four Volume Work: Topographical Positions of the Measurement Points of Electroacupuncture According to Voll. EAV Diagnosis of Eye Diseases, 15 New Measurement Points for Portions of the Eye, EAV Therapy for Eye Diseases, 5 New Approaches. Medizinisch Literarische Verlagesellschaft MBH, Uelzen, 1983.

Werbach MR, Murray MT. Botanical Influences on Illness. Tarzana, California: Third Line Press, 1994.

Whang S. Reverse Aging: Scientific Health Methods Easier and More Effective than Diet and Exercise (Siloam Enterprises, Englewood Cliffs, NJ, 1994).

Wurtman RJ, Baum MJ, and Potts JT. The Medical and Biological Effects of Light (The New York Academy of Sciences, New York, 1985).

About the Author

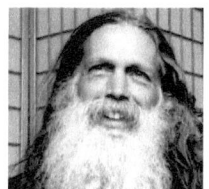

Rev. Dr. Glen Swartwout graduated Magna Cum Laude with honors in Environmental Earth Sciences and Chemistry from Dartmouth College, and received his doctorate at the top of his class in Vision Science with honors in Optics as well as Leadership, being inducted into both Beta Sigma Kappa and the Gold Key Honor Societies at the State University of New York in Manhattan, where he trained at the largest outpatient vision clinic in the world. He served as Editor, Vice President and President of the American Optometric Student Association serving 4000 international student doctor members. He is the author of over 50 professional papers, books, and software programs. His first professional office was in Tokyo, Japan.

Books

Refreshing Vision: Opening the Windows of the Soul

Healing Glaucoma

Healing Glaucoma

Cataract Solutions: Prevention & Reversal Via Accelerated Self-Healing

Macular Degeneration... ...Macular Regeneration

The Shire: Cultivating Your Future Self

Materia Medica: Vis Medicatrix Naturae

Electromagnetic Pollution Solutions

Biofields: The New Physics of Health

Nous Energy: Healing Power of the Pyramids

Additional writings

http://christiascelli.wordpress.com

http://doctorglen.wordpress.com

http://pahoasark.wordpress.com

http://selfgrowth.com/articles/user/240198

DVDs

A Clinical Theory of Everything

The Five Phases of Disease

The Five Phases of Healing

The Five Tissue Layers

The Five Levels of Regulation

The Five Elements of Spiritual Development

The Hard Question of Consciousness

The Arrow of Time

Additional contributions

Alternative Medicine, The Definitive Guide (contributor)

EPFX SCIO QXCI Quantum Xeroid Eclosion Consciousness Interface (contributor)

IBIS: Interactive BodyMind Information System (contributor)

Natural Eye Care, An Encyclopedia (co-author with Marc Grossman, O.D., L.Ac.)

Connect online

Website & Free E-zine signup: http://tryUnity.net

About.me: http://about.me/DrGlen

Healing Glaucoma

Facebook: http://facebook.com/DrSwartwout

LinkedIn:

http://www.linkedin.com/pub/Glen-Swartwout/10/902/5aa

Twitter: http://twitter.com/DoctorGlen

YouTube: http://youtube.com/DoctorGlen

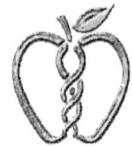

www.ingramcontent.com/pod-product-compliance
Lightning Source LLC
Chambersburg PA
CBHW021405170526
45164CB00002B/512